More Than You Can Handle

....

More Than You Can Handle

....

A Rare Disease, a Family in Crisis,
and the Cutting-Edge Medicine
That Cured the Incurable

MIGUEL SANCHO

Avery
an imprint of Penguin Random House
New York

AVERY

An imprint of Penguin Random House LLC
penguinrandomhouse.com

Most Avery books are available at special quantity discounts for bulk purchase for sales promotions, premiums, fund-raising, and educational needs. Special books or book excerpts also can be created to fit specific needs. For details, write SpecialMarkets@penguinrandomhouse.com.

Library of Congress Cataloging-in-Publication Data

Names: Sancho, Miguel, author.
Title: More than you can handle: A rare disease, a family in crisis, and the cutting-edge medicine that cured the incurable/ by Miguel Sancho.
Description: New York: Avery, an imprint of Penguin Random House, 2021. | Includes index.
Identifiers: LCCN 2020016997 (print) | LCCN 2020016998 (ebook) | ISBN 9780593085912 (hardcover) | ISBN 9780593085929 (ebook)
Subjects: LCSH: Sancho, Miguel. | Sancho, Sebastian, 2012—Health. | Chronic granulomatous disease—Patients—United States—Biography. | Parents of chronically ill children—United States—Biography.
Classification: LCC RJ387.C48 S26 2021 (print) | LCC RJ387.C48 (ebook) | DDC 618.92/970092 [B]—dc23
LC record available at https://lccn.loc.gov/2020016997
LC ebook record available at https://lccn.loc.gov/2020016998

Printed in the United States of America

1 3 5 7 9 10 8 6 4 2

Book design by Lorie Pagnozzi

To those who've had it tougher

Contents

Introduction

On the morning of December 22, 2003, a 6.6 magnitude earthquake struck the central coast of California near San Simeon. This was the most destructive quake to hit the United States since 1994, but thanks to modern construction standards and the seismic retrofitting of older buildings, only one building collapsed. The death toll was . . . two.

Just four days later, *another* 6.6 magnitude earthquake happened, this one near the ancient Iranian city of Bam. Most of the city's buildings were made of mud brick and did not comply with international earthquake regulations. Seventy percent of Bam's houses were destroyed. The death toll exceeded twenty-six thousand.

When we look inside ourselves and assess our own psychic sturdiness, the arrogant inclination is to believe we are constructed more like San Simeon than Bam—designed in anticipation of the worst our environment can dish out, made of sterner stuff. We all want to believe we have the ability to rise to the occasion of any crisis and perform nobly when the stakes are high. And the stakes get no higher than the life or death of a child. But what if fortitude is just another genetic trait like height or IQ, distributed normally on a bell curve, and what if you, like half of the population, are below average? Where will you find the strength to navigate your way through a black swan event, a once-in-a-lifetime disaster, without collapsing into a useless mold of Jell-O or perhaps managing to make things worse? What happens when God truly gives you more than you can handle?

For forty-two years, I never had to consider those questions. I never even had a real job—I made my living telling stories as a television news producer. It was my responsibility to find compelling stories and procure the necessary video to tell them. Then I wrote and edited scripts destined to be read by professionally attractive on-air talent, married to interesting pictures, and broadcast to the diminishing fraction of the public that chooses to spend its time watching commercial television—behavior we commended and encouraged. Sometimes my work won awards. Sometimes it got good ratings. Sometimes it did neither, but it always paid the bills.

Then something happened: I found myself thrust directly into the most amazing story I'd ever covered, one that blew my mind, broke my heart, and profoundly changed my life and many others', some at the molecular level. In 2012 my wife, Felicia, and I learned that our baby son, Sebastian, had a rare and deadly disease. It nearly killed him and destroyed our family in the process.

He is alive today, trundling off to school to master introductory subtraction, because he survived one of the most medically groundbreaking and emotionally harrowing procedures performed on earth—a pediatric bone marrow transplant (BMT).* The process required months of quarantine in a hermetically sealed transplant unit at Duke University Hospital, where doctors and researchers are taking giant steps—at an accelerating pace—in the fight against rare diseases once considered lethal. Families of children with these conditions come from all over the globe, rolling the dice that this lengthy, arduous, and highly uncertain procedure will save these patients' precious, origami-fragile lives. One of those children was Sebastian, who was born with a lethal

---

* Technically, his procedure was a "hematopoietic stem cell transplant" using umbilical cord blood, which gets explained later. For much of this book, I'll be using the more common term "bone marrow transplant," or BMT.

immune deficiency known as CGD (short for chronic granulomatous disease—no, I'd never heard of it either). By the time he left Duke he was not only cured, he'd been transformed into a wonder of science. This book is the story of that transformation and its impact on our family.

It is also something of a confession. It would be nice to be able to write that, over the course of Sebastian's illness and treatment, I met every challenge with selfless grace to save my darling child. Those are the heroic stories you read about in books like *Wonder*, or in the *Wired* article I read a while back about a Silicon Valley dad who spent his own millions to find a cure for his daughter's obscure genetic disorder. But not everyone confronted with this kind of challenge has an infinite reservoir of character or capital. Most of us are neither Mother Teresa nor Bill Gates.

The more common reality is that rare diseases frequently rip families apart. Divorce, substance abuse, depression, and bankruptcy are just a few of the horsemen riding in the slipstream of an apocalyptic diagnosis, and only a fraction of parents have the outstanding character and good fortune to avoid them all.

I was not among them. To the contrary, in the face of the biggest crisis of my life, I managed to derail my career, put my marriage on life support, get my family evicted and banned for life from the local Ronald McDonald House, and ruin a perfectly planned Make-A-Wish trip, to list a few of my greatest hits. When the wolf began blowing, I discovered my house was made of straw. Over time the stress disfigured my personality into a tangle of gnawing anxiety, insomnia, heavy drinking, frequent rage episodes at home and at work, and a depression resistant to numerous modalities of treatment (psychotherapy, meditation, medication, self-help books).

It would have been helpful if my emotional troubles manifested through socially sanctioned symptoms like fatigue or flattened affect.

Instead I found myself turning into a total dick. To be clear, the potential was always there—but my son's illness was, for me, an unstoppable catalyst, a defoliating agent that burned off what social graces I had and left a rather ugly stump. To call my nastiest behavior toxic masculinity would be an insult to both men and toxins, and I will state upfront that, for the sake of my family, I have not told *all* in this tell-all. The best thing I can say about myself during these years is that I never hit anybody.

And yet here we are, the lucky ones—children healthy, marriage intact, current on the mortgage. So many others have had it so much worse. That's why this book is also a thank-you note, a shout-out to a large cast of supporting characters that includes relatives, friends, doctors, nurses, other parents and patients, three different marriage counselors, a platoon of spiritual guides, Thomas the Tank Engine, a nanny from Medellín, and one rogue private investigator. Thanks to this community of generous souls—"angels," to use my wife's term—who guided our family through years of terror, pain, joy, and healing, we made it home in one piece. Thanks to them our story has a happy ending.

The book is also a valentine to science. As it happened, Sebastian's illness put him at the forefront of some of the most breathtaking innovations in modern medicine. Immunology is one of those fields advancing exponentially—its latest techniques border on science fiction—and as I immersed myself in it, I not only found cause for fascination but—for the first time in years—optimism, not just for my son but for the entire species. One might presume that in an age of rampant technophilia, such optimism would be commonplace and a book promoting it would be wholly unnecessary. And yet, antiscientific thinking abounds—from Hollywood stereotypes of scientists as heartless, power-mad Dr. Frankensteins meddling dangerously with nature to the persistence of pseudoscientific approaches regarding important matters of public health. (For personal reasons I harbor a singular scorn for the anti-vax movement, but this is only one of many examples.) If this book reduces, even microscopically, the world's burden of bullshit, I'll consider it a triumph.

We knew as we entered Unit 5200 at Duke University Hospital that it was a place where breathtaking, even buccaneering, medicine is practiced. What we didn't know is that it is also a place of immense love. This book is, at its root, about that—the intimate, incandescent, and tactile love generated by the claustrophobic gathering of individuals joined in the belief that human life is precious and worth preserving, even through radical and risky means. Inside that sterile womb, where the measure of time warps with each passing day, the infectious pathogens of the outside world—cruelty, pettiness, and prejudice—are kept on the other side of the doors with all the other lethal microbes. I've been to the Vatican, the Western Wall, and countless other places of worship. It was at my son's bedside where I came closest to God. For people like me, whose self-worth had been measured largely in the metrics of self-sufficiency and control, the experience provided a radical, transcendent (if slowly learned) lesson on the value of vulnerability. By the time Sebastian was fully healed, I'd also begun to reconcile many of the conflicts that had plagued my life so far—the struggles between science and spirituality, between order and chaos, between attachment and detachment.

In short, despite the catastrophic dimensions of the situation, and my own inexperience and ineptitude handling such matters, I was fortunate enough to find myself precisely where I needed to be, surrounded by the people who would motivate and inspire me to embrace these challenges, stare down my own demons, and—perhaps for the first time—truly behave like a grown man.

Felicia and I didn't get everything right. I got many things absolutely wrong. But we endured a harrowing experience, and we each developed our own methods for handling it: she called hers "the Five Fs of Life"; I called mine, half jokingly, "the Program." With any luck the lessons we learned will be of value to other parents who find themselves similarly overwhelmed by unforgiving circumstances. These moms and dads must become skilled quickly at what I term "parenting on the edge." This book is lastly a survival guide for these parents, a manual of dos and don'ts for anyone who has been tossed into extreme crisis and, regardless of their unsightly personal flaws, groped for a way to rise to the occasion—or at least limp across the finish line. This book will tell them what to expect from the unexpected.

A while back an old friend invited me to lunch, a big burly guy named Frank who also works in TV. I figured he wanted to talk shop, but I was wrong. He told me that he and his wife, Holly, hadn't slept in days because their son had just gotten some bad medical news. Immediate action was needed; full recovery was not guaranteed. They were lost; they needed guidance; and like any parents, they were torn up at a visceral level at the thought of their child suffering. For once I felt something I had to say might do someone a small measure of good. This book is for all the Franks and Hollys out there. There are millions of us.

Correction: billions of us. A curious thing happened as I began fact-checking the final version of this manuscript in early 2020—a new "rare" disease emerged on planet earth and ruthlessly proceeded to make itself conspicuously less rare. In a matter of weeks, the entire human species, which had no acquired immunity to COVID-19, has become intensely familiar with the fears and restrictions the immunocompromised and their families have lived with (and died with) for years. Immunology and epidemiology are the twin "it" sciences of the year. The distinctions between life in what we called "Hospitalworld" and "Healthyworld" have blurred, perhaps forever. For many in the community of the immunodeficient, inured to a lifestyle defined by germophobia, social distancing, and periods of full-blown quarantine, the attitude has been sympathetic but blunt: welcome to the club.

In our house, less than a mile outside the New Rochelle, New York, "containment area," the routines and precautions are familiar. We've simply reverted to Duke rules, and brought our old boxes of rubber gloves and masks up from the garage. Somehow we knew we'd be putting them to use one day.

There are two major differences this time around. On the downside, the global economy has ground to a halt with a suddenness that has been as surreal as it is violent, and the crisis has exposed cracks and inadequacies in the health care system which—fingers crossed—will be thoroughly and permanently addressed before the human toll escalates from the obscene to the incomprehensible. On the upside, we count it as a blessing to be more concerned about the survival of our aged parents than our youngest child.

By the time this book is published, it could either be precisely in sync with the times, or it could be entirely irrelevant. But, as many of our friends have approached us for advice in the past weeks, it feels right to pass along some practical lessons we learned the hard way. If you read like I do, you may never finish this book, but if you can just make it to the end of this introduction, you'll get the main takeaways for the Age of COVID.

First, understand that the psychological aspects of the experience are as real and in some ways as dangerous as the biological threat. It doesn't take much time for your mind to start playing dirty tricks on you. I spent six years in a mental state dominated by some combination of fear, anger, and sadness. The havoc wreaked on every aspect of my life was profound. I am highly skeptical that hell exists after death; I am equally positive it exists on earth—we create it whenever we let extreme negativity define our reality. If you find yourself slipping in that direction, do whatever it takes to redirect yourself—I mean everything from meditation to medication to exercise to therapy to prayer and whatever else you want to try. Most of all—make sure you get regular sleep by any means necessary. Otherwise both your brain chemistry and immune system can deteriorate dramatically.

Second, as noted above, quarantine with close family doesn't have to be just an experience of extreme anxiety; it can also be an experience of deep, intimate love. Think of it as mandated quality time—time to block out the countless distractions and explore new possibilities in your closest relationships. This can be something as simple as enjoying a few rounds of Just Dance 2020 with a tween daughter, as I did for the first time this weekend. Whenever you're spending time with people you love, your time is never wasted.

Finally, try to keep some sense of perspective. I am not suggesting we ignore the directives or pooh-pooh the gravity of a massive public health crisis, nor am I advocating callousness toward the most vulnerable. But I am suggesting that the ideal of perfect safety can be a pernicious and destructive myth. Risk is everywhere; life is more random and unfair than any of us can truly understand and stay sane. It can be wonderful; it is always finite.

While Sebastian was in transplant I had a memorable conversation with a stress management nurse clinician at Duke Hospital. He'd seen forty thousand patients over the course of his career, quite a few of whom didn't make it. He said he'd known twenty-five-year-old cystic fibrosis patients who'd reconciled themselves to their mortality with much more equanimity than some eighty-year-old cancer patients. The young CF patients had accepted the reality that they didn't have much time; they'd made the most of it; they'd worked past the anger, sadness, and fear and found a reservoir of natural nobility that guided them through each successive emergency, right till the end. "It's not age that prepares you for death," he told me, "it's how you live."

I've been ambivalent about organized religion my entire life. It can veer easily into superstition and self-righteousness, but it can also provide a uniquely helpful vocabulary to cope with life's greatest challenges. I lack the moral authority to invoke the power of this language, but with the human race trembling in fear of deadly infection as I write, allow me, just this once: peace be with you.

Westchester County, NY
March 2020

More Than You Can Handle

....

Part 1

Wars Without Guns

May 2012–March 2016

Chapter 1

Please Fasten Your Seat Belts

Daddy: a touching term of endearment, an exalted job title, and presently—*"Daddy!!"*—a blaring distress signal.

The scene: Delta flight 6056, a claustrophobic regional jet as tight on legroom as food options, en route from LaGuardia to Raleigh-Durham, North Carolina. Me in seat 12C, splitting attention between the *Sky* magazine crossword and my seven-year-old daughter, Lydia, seated next to me and enraptured by the images on the laminated safety card. Two rows back and across the aisle, my wife, Felicia, and our three-year-old boy, Sebastian. The captain had just announced our impending descent in his best *The Right Stuff* voice of practiced professional calm. The Fasten Seat Belt sign was on.

"Daddy!!!!!"—my wife using my domestic moniker, her voice almost a Jamie Lee Curtis horror movie scream the second time. I whipped my head around, spilling a plastic cup of Diet Coke into my lap as I fumbled for some way to help. I turned just in time to witness a small fountain of vomit, the tapioca pudding variety, spewing from our son's discolored lips onto Felicia's blouse. My wife looked at me with her big brown eyes, silent, blinking back panic. Then she tilted her head down to the convulsing child prostrate in her lap, his head rolled back, lifeless. An economy class pietà.

"His head is *burning up!*" she announced to the cabin, just as he went

3

into some kind of seizure or febrile spasm. I didn't know the difference, which made it all the worse.

There may be circumstances less hospitable to medical emergencies, but aside from some vivid memories of the aftermath of the 2010 Haiti earthquake, none came to mind as I remained strapped, seated, and upright, lifted my arm, and pressed the flight attendant call button—a profile in impotence.

Lydia, preternaturally serene, tugged my sleeve and pointed to the safety card's diagram of a water landing. "What if *this* happens?" she mused with wonder. I shut my eyes and conjured an image of Sully Sullenberger, mentally beseeching his avuncular, disembodied face for guidance. *Waddya think, Sully? How would you handle this one?*

The image pursed its mustachioed lips and shook its head.

Like any disaster movie, this trip had begun as an exercise in quotidian blandness. Booked on Expedia months in advance, it was conceived as the latest in a long series of medical tourism weekends for our family. Three and a half years prior, Sebastian had been diagnosed with CGD, an extremely rare, often lethal immune deficiency with which he'd been born. The diagnosis ripped through our lives, careers, and relationships like a twister through a Missouri trailer park, and we'd spent every day since in some degree of distress—sometimes quiet, often loud—as we struggled to keep him out of danger, out of the ICU, out of the grave. Vacations were one of several aspects of our lives that had been radically recolored. Now if we ventured outside our domestic safe zone, the destination was usually one of the country's top children's hospitals as we pursued an Arthurian quest for a cure.

That quest had led us to North Carolina. Today's itinerary included this Delta flight to Durham, a rented Dodge Caravan, and an appointment at Duke University Hospital for a meet and greet with the team at the Pediatric Blood and Marrow Transplant Unit, possibly the only people on earth who could rid Sebastian of his disease. The transplantation procedure is among the most grueling in modern medicine, so before we committed, the doctors wanted to walk us through the process, show us the facilities, run some preliminary diagnostic tests, and lay out a timetable for when we'd move down from our Westchester County home to begin a yearlong "journey"—the preferred euphemism for "ordeal." If we had time, over the weekend we'd explore local housing and school options. Simple enough.

Any travel plan involving a chronically ill kid is risky, but Sebastian had been doing so well in the past few months that Felicia and I summoned enough optimism to forgo travelers' insurance. I even had the audacity to snag two tickets to a Billy Joel show at Madison Square Garden earlier that week. Neither of us is a huge fan—to be frank I'd rather get a Brazilian wax than endure a performance of "We Didn't Start the Fire"—but this was a rare opportunity for us to have a proper date night and recapture some of our pre-kids, pre-diagnosis frisson.

Fate put those plans in the shredder. Five days before our scheduled departure Sebastian came down with a mysterious fever, accompanied by a nagging cough. For most parents of a kid that age, that's a plain-vanilla health issue. Just dose the kid with acetaminophen, crank up the bedroom humidifier, and wait three days for the clouds to part.

Not so with parents of the immunodeficient, who regard fever and cough much as ancient Roman diviners evaluated an abnormal sheep liver or a statue struck by lightning. Bad omens. The first sign of symptoms triggered a response routine that, while well practiced enough to be second nature, was still sufficiently stressful to make our innards do the lambada as we awaited an accurate diagnosis. Calls to the pediatrician, blood draws, cultures, chest X-rays. All the while that merciless cough, a periodic honk in the throat mixed with the hideous sound of mucus whipping around deep in the lungs, marked time through sleepless nights—the body's version of a smoke alarm's low-battery chirp.

The timing simply sucked. I was on the tail end of a labor-intensive project at work—I was a television news producer and late nights of kung pao chicken and 1 a.m. Uber pickups had become frequent enough to pass for a lifestyle. That week my extended obligations at the office meant stiffing Felicia with the lion's share of the parental responsibility. She'd cut back on her professional life as a PR consultant to become Sebastian's primary caregiver years ago, but despite her expertise a situation like this was tough to manage alone. An hour tending to a sick child passes like three hours of regular life; after four days the experience is a masonry grinder for the mind.

The fever oscillated between 102 and 104, but it never broke. A doctor at a nearby hospital eyeballed an X-ray, ruled out pneumonia, and decreed we had nothing but a run-of-the-mill virus on our hands. In theory we could manage that, but as the symptoms persisted, Felicia's customary suspicion of the local sawbones prompted a call down to the experts at Duke for advice. Should we proceed as planned with the trip or postpone until Sebastian was in better shape to travel?

"They didn't hesitate," she reported over the phone as I sat amid a pile of scripts on my office desk. "They said he needs to get down there right away. Whatever he's got, they can handle it best if he's there."

"And . . . "—indecision decelerating the pace of my speech—"what are *you* thinking?"

"We need to go. Something's not right. *I know my child.*"

That last bit was code for "Don't question me," a declaration of steely resolve that, in this instance among many others, likely saved our son's life.

The next morning our plane was wheels up on schedule and it appeared fortune had granted us a respite. Sebastian's fever dipped to 101, not great but tolerable, and his affect was on the upswing as he peered out the window, digging the g-force of the takeoff. Rikers Island, then the Archie Bunker blocks of Queens and the rest of New York, receded behind gray cotton candy clouds. But somewhere over the Chesapeake Bay the shit hit the fan. Fever, barf, spasms, terror.

Our worst-case scenario was now, indeed, the case. It looked like our son was infected with an unknown pathogen against which he was defenseless, and it was spreading throughout his lungs. Most people don't give it much thought, but the biology of infection is as scary as it is gross—another life-form invades the body, feeding off it parasitically as it grows and multiplies. Unchecked, the microbes chew away at healthy tissue, eventually commandeering so much space and resources to trigger organ failure. The body—in this case our three-year-old child's beautiful little body, clothed in a Thomas the Tank Engine sweatshirt and shod in Velcro-strap sneakers—literally gets eaten alive . . . from the inside.

Sporting an expression that somehow conveyed both kindness and exasperation, a flight attendant worked her way up the aisle in response to my call. I noticed that Sebastian had wet himself. The spilled Diet Coke in my lap made a matching mark on my slacks—the shape of a gerrymandered Massachusetts congressional district. I reached for a napkin and covered my crotch as I asked her what could be done. There was some first-aid equipment stowed in the rearmost overhead baggage compartments, she explained, but while the plane was in its final descent it was illegal to access it. We were on our own. The one option was to radio ground control to have an ambulance intercept us on the runway if this was indeed a matter of life and death.

Was it? How the fuck was I supposed to know?

Big decision, little information, even less time. I did what came naturally: I froze.

"Let's give it a few minutes," Felicia said from her seat as she wiped vomit from her blouse with some Huggies baby wipes and stuffed them into the air-sickness bag. "Just . . . give it a few minutes. And pray . . ."

The flight attendant bestowed a sympathetic pat on my arm and worked her way back to her jump seat. I faked a smile at Lydia as she pointed to a carpet of North Carolina oak and hickory trees that had just come into view as our glide path brought the Embraer 170 down from the asphalt sky. The fuselage shuddered from mild turbulence. The captain came on the intercom once more and, in a voice more firm than gentle this time, explained the nonnegotiability of the FAA requirement to stow all tray tables. Apparently a recalcitrant Tar Heel six rows up had her own opinions on the matter.

My son was whimpering; my wife was weeping; my daughter was elsewhere. I gripped the armrest. Instead of praying, I tried to remember how it had all come to this. . . .

It is the immutable duty of any storyteller to recruit a measure of sympathy for the tale's protagonists. With Felicia, that's a layup. An only child, Felicia grew up in the distinctly middle-class Chicago neighborhood of Albany Park.

Her mom was a free-spirited Canadian idealist; her dad, a soft-spoken Appalachian man who'd made his way from the mountains of West Virginia to the big city and a union job on the floor of a large toy manufacturer. Their house had Glen Campbell on the turntable and the Holy Bible on the nightstand. Her dad stayed true to his rural roots, growing berries, beans, and even corn in the backyard, referring to his garage as "the barn." Felicia heard him saying his prayers each night, thanking God for his home and his family.

From that upbringing emerged a well-traveled, outspoken, and independent woman, possessed of what her mother's Finnish forebears called *sisu*, their word for perseverance or grit. At least that's how she appeared from the outside. By her own account, she also harbored deep insecurities and a need to prove to herself and to the world that she was good enough.

Tall, slender, brunette—she made a great Olive Oyl or Morticia Addams at Halloween. Teenage rebellion for her meant cranking Erasure and New Order, hanging out with dangerous boys, digging the head rush of Djarum clove cigarettes.

On the strength of her own brains and willpower, she'd gone to college and graduate school, lived and worked in Prague for three years, and cultivated a keen taste for fashion and opera. She'd moved to D.C. and launched a promising career as a print journalist, writing for online editions of the *Washington Post* and the *Wall Street Journal*. A stint as an online tech columnist left her feeling empty, and, compelled by an innate desire to help others, she moved to Manhattan to try to make a difference post-9/11. She started volunteering for victims' family efforts and landed a job with an international PR firm.

We met through mutual 9/11 connections and commenced a classic New York love affair. (This was not the first time something beautiful blossomed against a background of crisis and destruction, and for us it would not be the last.) Within months I edged out a wolf pack of other suitors and convinced her to marry me—perhaps our mutual appreciation of inane puns sealed the deal—and we looked forward to starting a family. In the meantime she'd launched her own boutique public relations consultancy. By any measure, she'd done well for herself. Moreover, she was funny, humble, and if anything, too considerate of others. By no means was she a saint, but her imperfections were easy to overlook. She is the hero of this story.

As for myself? I can say this: I've tried. Tried to be a principled person, a loyal friend, a good employee, a devoted husband and father. My ambitions were precisely this: to have a family I loved and a job I didn't hate. But along the way some things I expected to be easy turned out to be hard; some things that were supposed to be hard turned out to be easy. Still others turned out to be *too* easy. In its own way that can be a curse.

A proud Gen Xer, I was born to a Costa Rican mother and a Nuyorican father in Lawrence, Kansas, of all places, while they were both completing graduate studies in chemistry at KU. I grew up in Kansas City, Missouri, as they pursed unglamorous but noble teaching careers, which afforded them ample downtime to raise me and my younger sister. Identified as a precocious student with an acumen for math and science, I was guided toward a career in medicine.

Blessed with an exquisite education at the nation's best schools, I chose to turn my back on hard science and pursue a degree in humanities. That's what the cool kids seemed to be doing. (Shortly thereafter, the uncool kids would become dot-com billionaires. Count that as one of my many questionable decisions with life-changing repercussions. In a corner of my mind there's a trophy case full of them.)

After college and a risible attempt to make it as a musician in New York, I essentially stumbled into a career in television journalism. The pace and variety of the profession harmonized with my personality and I made a good living, met a wonderful woman, bought a Manhattan apartment, and started making babies. I hadn't been raised rich, and many of my friends made *real* money, but I certainly qualified as comfortable.

Better yet, I'd been truly pampered by fate. After forty years on the planet I had yet to confront a problem out of which I couldn't talk, work, or pay my way. Tragedy rained from the sky daily, in sizes small (newsworthy murders and frauds) and big (9/11, Operation Iraqi Freedom, the Great Recession). But tragedy was something that happened to *other* people—the people whose suffering was, in fact, the raw material my colleagues and I mined and refined for a living.

In short, I paid my mortgage primarily as a chronicler of others' misfortune, albeit a conscientious one. Spending so much time rooting through the detritus of human troubles should have taught me that one day my own number might be called and fortified me for that shock. Sadly, that's not how it played. After a lifetime walking between the raindrops, I'd come to expect everything to work out, especially with my offspring.

It all fell into place. Felicia and I moved into a two-bedroom co-op apartment on 49th Street and First Avenue. The neighborhood was so dowdy I convinced myself it bestowed a reverse cool, our building's only amenity. After a smooth pregnancy, Felicia gave birth to our beloved Lydia on July 3, 2008, so close to Independence Day we considered naming her America. (No apologies—this was the heyday of baby Brooklyns and Madisons.) I promoted my Colombian housekeeper, Mercedes, to official nannydom. Mountains of baby stuff and gigabytes of pictures ensued. The works.

Adjusting to the demands and sacrifices wasn't a snap—to be frank I had a hard time surrendering all the indulgences of our lives as DINKs (double income no kids). But through trial (hers) and error (mostly mine) Felicia and I made it work. It helped that Lydia was such a worthy subject of devotion. Intensely alert, precociously verbal, incorruptibly innocent. Every father loves his daughter like he's never loved another female, so feel free to impugn my objectivity, but—swear to God—we'd be waiting at a bus stop and hear passersby exclaim, "Look at that *perfect baby!*" At five months we took her to Chicago, and at the Art Institute a group of Japanese tourists turned away from Seurat's *A Sunday on La Grande Jatte* and started taking pictures of *her.* Bottom line—had we subjected this child to the cruelties of the infant modeling industry she could have gone Gerber.

By the time I hit forty I had ample evidence to believe the trajectory of our lives would be one continuous ascent—Lydia was two and a half, gorgeous, bright, and adorable in proportions measureless to man. Aside from some sporadic and treatable asthma, her health was stellar. We couldn't get enough of her. With a trouble-free child, parenting is as invigorating as it is exhausting. The world grants you license to be a kid again yourself, a passport to a universe of fun stuff off-limits to any childless adult who doesn't want to look like a perv going to the circus, climbing jungle gyms, or vacationing at theme parks. You can eat pizza and cake at the half-dozen birthday parties you're suddenly invited to every month. The holidays, no longer a season of cynical inebriation, morph into a month of nonstop enchantment. Parenting *rejuvenates* in the most literal sense of the word.

By 2011 we were hungry for seconds. Felicia got pregnant again just as I got a promotion at work, and we were delighted to learn we'd be having a boy. I was to be the head of a classic "millionaire's family."

High on life, I found myself in a delivery room at St. Luke's-Roosevelt hospital, as it was then known, on May 1, 2012. Outside in the waiting area it was the D train at rush hour; inside the delivery room was as tranquil as an ashram. The prenatal diagnostics, including a full battery of amnio tests for genetic defects, had been an uninterrupted series of thumbs-ups, and now Felicia, fully epiduraled and Lamazed, was making the final push.

The ob-gyn performed admirably, though I don't remember his name. In those days, I had a habit of forgetting doctors' names because, like many American men under fifty, I basically regarded them as auto mechanics—I respected their profession but I deemed them little more than service providers, my time spent with them a necessary nuisance at best. How long would this take, how much would it cost?—my curiosity about their craft extended no further. When this guy delivered Sebastian without incident I resisted the urge to hand him a tip.

"Oh, you're so beautiful!" a nurse proclaimed as Sebastian arrived, aced his Apgar, and weighed in at eight pounds, nine ounces. I assumed they say that to all the babies, though vernix-coated newborns scarcely resemble Michelangelo's cherubim. But the nurses have their own standards of beauty. "Just look at the symmetry of his head," intoned another, "a perfect dome!" I got what they meant a few hours later when Sebastian was wheeled off for his first bath. The kid just ahead of him in line had an angelic face, but the back of his cranium was oddly cubic, a hairy lunch box. Once again, I was the lucky one. The hospital had a professional photographer on call to take some high-end happy snaps before we were discharged. The four of us were literally the portrait of domestic bliss.

We were experienced parents by now, yet as we carried our newborn son into our apartment we noted what a remarkable thing it is that the state simply allows people to take babies home a mere two days after delivery. New York requires three hundred hours of course work and two examinations before it grants a license to style hair, yet it allows pretty much anyone to become a parent with little guidance and zero supervision. One day a dwelling houses three people; the next, regardless of mom and dad's aptitude or preparedness, there's a fourth, infinitely needy and vulnerable. It's a wonder so many of them survive. "Doesn't it feel like someone from the Department of Health is going to knock on the door and say, 'Okay, your time's up, we need him back'?" Felicia joked.

It was false modestly—in truth we were supremely confident in our parenting skills. Like most couples in twenty-first-century developed countries, we planned to have fewer children than past generations, but we fully expected them to be perfect. Between our genes and our diligence, we would nature-and-nurture them straight to the top. Given that standard, it qualified as a serious concern when we noticed later that week that Sebastian's ears were ever so slightly pointed, a bit like a bat's. On the second or third of several standard visits to our pediatrician's office in the early weeks, I broached the subject. Was there anything to be concerned about? Anything that could be done?

"You have no idea the kind of issues other parents are dealing with, amigo," the attending physician said. "The shit I see every day. Birth defects, catastrophic delivery mishaps, organ failure. How about this—you get the fuck out of here, go home, and thank God for your good fortune."

No. That's not what she really said. Those are the words I'm using to verbalize the sulfuric disdain I detected in her eyes as she calmly replied, "If you're really troubled by the ears, we can talk about cosmetic surgery, but I wouldn't advise it."

I understood both her words and her eyes. We left in chastened silence and went back to our cozy apartment to bask in the enchantment only a newborn can provide. We were truly blessed.

Were we ripe for a karmic ass kicking? Did we deserve what was to come? Shackled inside countless sleepless nights, stomachs churning and minds ablaze with worry and guilt, Felicia and I would chew over that thought for years. It was only after we'd met other parents who'd been dealt the same hand—humble and dignified people who yearned for nothing more than the contentment of a healthy family—that I could find solace in a memorable line of Eastwood dialogue: "Deserve's got nothin' to do with it. . . ."

Chapter 2

Welcome to Hospitalworld

....

"Hay problema con el niño." Mercedes, our nanny, had a distinctive look of solemn worry on her face, a look earned the hard way during her adolescence in Medellín. *"Tiene fiebre todavía."*

A fever had lingered for three days. Mercedes was certain something was wrong. Something unusual. She'd raised five kids of her own and had a reliable sixth sense about these things, though in this case two would have sufficed had I been using them properly.

Instead, I was clinging to the belief that my son, simply by being mine, was a strapping super-infant who would register off the charts in every metric that mattered—from height percentile to IQ. From the outset, I'd dismissed his illness as a nothingburger. I'd been minimizing medical matters successfully for forty-one years, and besides, *What to Expect the First Year* provided enough soothing advice to justify a blasé attitude: babies can get fevers and they run hotter than adults. So when Sebastian woke up on June 27, 2012, with a temperature of 100.6, I figured it was par for the course for a seven-week-old.

Following both the book's and doctors' orders over the phone, we'd administered acetaminophen and cool baths. That seemed to do the trick for a while, but every eight hours the fever boomeranged back, hotter than ever. Sebastian expressed his misery with the nasal "*eh-HEH, eh-HEH*" plea that's drawn countless new parents cribside with consternation. You could set your watch by it.

On the third morning, minutes after Mercedes issued her warning, Sebastian spat up a green-blue barf, re-creating Monet's water lilies on the chest of his onesie. Felicia hit the mute button on my bullshit and banished me to the office; she was headed to the pediatrician's. One of those Upper East Side medical suites nested into the first floor of a luxury residential building, the place's address, we'd been assured, was synonymous with superior care.

Two hours later I was standing behind my elevated, ergonomically enlightened desk when the call came.

"Take him to the *ER?!*" I blurted into the speakerphone, though the pediatrician, Dr. Gary Edelstein, had spoken with perfect elocution and there are few terms in the English language less obscure than *ER*. Edelstein, a casually fit and exceedingly affable doctor who could have been a recurring side character on *Seinfeld*, calmly repeated himself and explained that, yes, this was no longer a run-of-the-mill baby fever.

He'd ordered a blood workup at the office, what's known as a complete blood count, or a CBC—one of many basic medical terms I'd never needed to know until now. This marked the first time Sebastian's veins were pierced for a blood draw. The desperate, terrified scream the needle precipitated would eventually become as familiar to Felicia and me as the opening chord from "A Hard Day's Night," but we'd never get used to it. I've poked my nose into many a parenting book. None of them tell you how to watch your child suffer.

The blood work came back with a coded message: "WBC 22"—five simple characters in eight-point font on a piece of paper. To an ignoramus like myself it was gibberish; to any medical professional it was as familiar and troublesome as a ground proximity warning is for an airline pilot. Sebastian's white blood cell count (WBC) was sky-high, a flashing red signal his immune system had been triggered and was now in overdrive—he'd acquired an infection and was trying to fight it. A WBC of 22 was rare for a child that young and well cared for. My boy was indeed off the charts. Just not in the ways I'd envisioned.

I assumed an "Rx for oral ABX" (a prescription for antibiotics in medical records speak) would be an adequate remedy. I assumed wrong. With a baby less than two months old there's a chance the infection is a sepsis-induced meningitis, which can be fatal. The tests to determine that require a spinal tap, and by the time those results come back the infection can have already spread to the brain. Delay can mean death. The uniform standard of care is to hospitalize the patient immediately, perform the spinal tap, initiate intravenous antibiotics even before the results come back to get ahead of a worst-case scenario, and hold the patient for observation.

This was the first time the words "dead baby" had ever crossed my mind, and I paid them scant regard. This had the ring of one of those abundance-of-caution responses from the government in the face of a chatter-driven national security scare. Memories of taping Xs on my apartment windows in 2002 after Tom Ridge put the county on orange alert pirouetted through my mind as I eloped from work and made my way crosstown to the emergency room of New York–Presbyterian, the East Side hospital near to our apartment with which Edelstein was affiliated.

There are two kinds of parents in this world—those who've taken a child to an emergency room, and those who haven't. Regardless of what brings you there—a swallowed Tide pod, a hot-stove burn, or an undiagnosed mystery illness like ours—the sense of fear and failure is transformative, puncturing whatever arrogant self-image you might have harbored as an ideal mommy or daddy. The judgment-free manner of the staff notwithstanding, the irreducible reality hangs on your neck like a millstone: something has gone wrong on your watch. The state may have let you amateurs take that newborn home, but now trained professionals must intervene. It's official: the situation is more than you can handle.

After completing a ream of paperwork, we spent hours in a curtained examination bay, watching baby videos on a TV mounted in the corner. An IV went in and more blood came out as a bedroom up on the pediatric unit was prepped. Felicia and I labored to make small talk.

It was dinnertime before Sebastian was wheeled past the benevolent smiles on the portrait of Mr. and Mrs. Sanford Weill, the billionaire banker-philanthropist for whom the pediatric unit is named. The portrait was a mild sedative—if a Wall Street titan put his name on the place, how bad could it be? In any case, we'd been assured this was all just precautionary. Assuming the sepsis tests were negative and the fever broke, we'd be heading home in two days. Likely this was just some viral infection.

That evening we felt it for the first time—the dramatic recalibrations of time, priorities, and social status that occur when you enter what we'd come to call Hospitalworld. In our normal lives, we were somebodies. We had control of our schedules. We were endowed with a measure of authority at work. We had considerable say in any decision affecting our family. And were certainly free to leave any place we went at a moment's notice. None of that was true here.

Neither of us could be called a control freak, but everyone needs a modicum of order and predictability in their lives just to function. Quite rapidly, that order was ceding ground to the forces of chaos. This new sense of helplessness was palpable. For a male head of household, the word is "emasculating." As Sebastian fell asleep, I leaned into Felicia's ear and whispered, "I really want to get the uckfay out of erehay."

We tag-teamed the days and nights, one of us sleeping on the room's full-length couch while the other went home to relieve Mercedes and care for Lydia. Our daughter was quizzical but calm—"Why's Sebastian at the hospital? Are you giving him back?"—but whatever was behind this mysterious disturbance, she assumed it would rectify itself shortly, as had every other ripple in her short, happy life.

She was right. The spinal tap and a host of other tests came back negative. An ECG revealed a perfect "cardio rhythmic silhouette." Two days later we were discharged, and as I struggled to collapse Sebastian's stroller into the back of a cab—mastery of our particular model required an engineering degree—I truly felt this would turn out to be nothing but a brief inconvenience, a pit stop at the auto mechanic.

The fever returned that night—at 3 a.m. Sebastian spiked 102 and was clearly suffering. Tylenol barely nudged the thermometer. Over the next few days, as our prior confidence sank into a quicksand of creeping fear, Edelstein confirmed that the WBC was still at 20. He had no clear reason why.

Our "diagnostic odyssey"—an actual term among the rare-disease crowd—had begun. Edelstein ordered another battery of tests to rule out everything from pneumonia to a thyroid condition called Hashimoto's disease. A low iron count—anemia—had us in the office of a hematologist. His tests yielded nothing but further bewilderment. During our follow-up visit, as he shifted his eyes from the lab results to Sebastian's face, he could only mutter, "Well, *something's* going on in there."

It was now July 6, ten days since the fever first arrived, and it showed no sign of abating. Edelstein ordered us back to Hospitalworld, and upon readmission it was clear we had entered a realm of medical mystery. Fresh tests for common bacteria and viruses yielded precisely bubkes. Suddenly a buffet of more exotic explanations was spread out before us—a barely detectable spot on the chest X-ray could or could not be pneumonia. Legionnaires' disease entered the discussion, since

Sebastian's crib at home was near a unit air conditioner; the corresponding urine antigen test was ordered. And why was his left leg suddenly moving less? A neurologist arrived to opine on the matter.

This interdepartmental clown car quickly grew tiresome. The rising number of experts assigned to the task tracked with our eroding faith in their aggregate efficacy. Their swelling confusion was scary enough—when a dozen doctors don't know what to do, it's hard to remain calm, but soon our fear gave way to annoyance. Every two hours another new white coat shuffled in and asked us to recite Sebastian's complete medical history from the beginning like ancient Greek oral poets who passed down the *Iliad* before the alphabet was invented.

The notion that we, parents in distress, were being relied upon to recall every detail and test result, any datum of which could mean the difference between diagnosis and misdiagnosis, was supremely aggravating. "Don't you guys have iPads or something where all this information could be stored?" I snapped. We later learned this was part of the hospital's training regimen—dispatching young residents into the rooms to get hands-on experience interacting with patients and families.

Sebastian himself wasn't aggrieved by any of this. The hospital records from that date describe a "well-appearing child." If anything, he just appeared lost, overwhelmed by all these other people around him. Where were "his people," as one nurse put it—mommy and daddy? It's fun to think of infants as Boss Babies, capable of coherent reasoning, even cunning. But consider how truly unformed nine-week-old babies are. Not even out of the so-called fourth trimester, scarcely familiar with their own bodies, oblivious to the world beyond their immediate range of vision, still unacquainted with concepts of the future or the past. Not *really* complete people in the way we usually conceive of personhood.

Many never get to become complete people. Babies have been dying for millennia, often for sudden and unexplained reasons. This notion that *every baby must live* is a recent contrivance among developed nations. I'd grown up believing my own mother was the youngest of ten kids in a large Costa Rican family. In fact, she is the youngest of eleven—one of her siblings, a baby girl, died of an unspecified infection at six months. Her death was a tragedy but not an anomaly. A mere two generations ago it was commonly understood and accepted: *some infants just don't make it.* That's one of the reasons people had so many— to hedge their bets.

It's also why parents of seriously sick newborns often try to adopt a posture of emotional detachment. One mother we'd later meet recalled the moment her son first got sick. At seven weeks he'd acquired a fungal infection that had severely ulcerated his intestines. He was medevaced to a regional intensive care unit for emergency surgery, the doctors using every available vein in his arms and legs to infuse lifesaving meds. They quickly ran out and had to use a vein in his head. Despite those efforts the odds were long; the doctors told the mother they'd never seen anyone survive an infection that bad.

"When they told me that, I didn't want to go back into the ICU, I didn't want to see my son again," she told me. "I couldn't believe I could love someone this much and God was going to take him away. And if that was going to happen, I didn't want to love him any more than I already did." Eventually she came around, but her father went into a shell. "He didn't even want to touch the baby. He simply couldn't face the imminent death of his grandson. He checked out. *This is not real.*"

We were grappling with similar feelings. My initial nonchalance had vanished like a drawing on a shaken Etch A Sketch. Now the words "dead baby" were ringing in my head. "I cannot believe this is happening," said Felicia, mostly to herself, as we sat vigilantly in Sebastian's room awaiting news. Scouring my memory for some source of reassurance, I quoted some TV doctor—probably Sanjay Gupta—remarking about American medicine: "We're not that good at making people healthy, but we're *really good* at keeping people alive." The quip was uttered half jokingly; now I needed it to be true.

"And then . . . do you know what happened? A *miracle!*" (F. Murray Abraham in *Amadeus*.) The fever simply disappeared. No medicine required, no medical intervention at all. On Tuesday, I'd been wondering if we'd soon be planning a funeral. On Thursday, we were sent home with no guidance other than to keep Sebastian on a new hypoallergenic formula and to call back if symptoms returned. He had an annoying and persistent diaper rash, but that was so minor and common it scarcely merited mention.

The angel of death had tickled our baby's chin and moved on. As we trundled back into our apartment, Felicia and I hugged each other. Maybe we even high-fived. We'd been tested. We'd passed. If there was any justice in this universe, we wouldn't revisit Hospitalworld until my first heart attack.

Get back on track, I said to myself, like so many parents derailed temporarily by a child's medical emergency. *Just . . . get back on track. . . .*

On the morning of August 16, I was on diaper duty. After wiping Sebastian's impossibly cute buns, I noticed something odd: a strange, light-red bump near his rectum on the left side. When I pressed it, he cried out in pain. I had to head to work so I told Felicia about it and she said she'd call Edelstein immediately. I figured it was just swelling related to the diaper rash. Maybe that's just what I wanted it to be.

A few fretful hours later I was at the office when Felicia called from the pediatrician's. The problem itself wasn't too serious, Edelstein explained on speaker. Sebastian's bump was a perirectal abscess, a subcutaneous lump likely caused by a bacterial infection. "These things are common in babies with diaper rash," he explained. "Some small fissure happens in the irritated skin and it gets infected with bacteria from the poop. It's no biggie, especially since he has no fever, but the infection has to be treated promptly."

As the "get back on track" reflex kicked in I imagined this meant the application of some antibiotic ointment, a prescription-level bacitracin.

No, he said. Sebastian needs surgery.

Disbelief. "Full surgery? With general anesthesia?"

Yes.

"Intubation?"

Yes.

"Readmission to the hospital?"

Yes.

A normal, adult abscess is typically handled in a GP's office and treatment is completed in a matter of minutes. A simple application of iodine-based antiseptic on the affected area, a minor incision to puncture the skin, and then a drainage of pus and cleansing of the wound. Basically, a glorified zit popping.

With babies it's different. They won't hold steady long enough to make sure the incision is executed properly, and because this abscess was near the rectum they needed Sebastian fully sedated.

All of this was explained to me by a pediatric surgeon I'm calling Susanna Mossberg as we sat in the now-familiar ER later that day, waiting for Sebastian to be rolled into an operating room. She'd done hundreds of these, she explained, and the rate of success was extremely high. The entire procedure shouldn't last more than fifteen minutes.

They let me put on a paper body suit, head covering, and mask to accompany him into the OR. A circle of similarly attired strangers was assembled around a table outfitted with a baby-sized headrest and restraints. I gasped quietly under my mask. Resisting the feeling of powerlessness, I asked everyone their names. "Stay focused now," I said cheerily, knowing this was probably their fifth or sixth procedure of the day. "No mistakes allowed!" This was my lame way of telegraphing that I'd sue with a vengeance if anything went wrong. They nodded, said some nice things, and let me hold Sebastian's hand as they put a plastic mask on his face to put him under. They'd coated the edge of the mask with a red gel. It made the gas taste like strawberry.

His hand went limp in mine. Then they made it clear it was time for me to go, and for the first time since he'd been conceived, our baby was no longer under our supervision.

Get back on track.

Felicia and I sat in the waiting room, shell-shocked. Only yesterday all had been well. "Why is this happening to him?" Felicia lamented, gnashing her teeth at the evil unfairness. The doctors had resisted making a connection between this abscess and the previous mystery fever. Just a short series of unfortunate events, they'd said—"This just happens to some children." We chose to believe them.

Half an hour later the heavy automatic OR doors opened with a *shnnnshhh* and Mossberg the surgeon emerged, expressionless, and told us all had gone well. Sebastian was heading to the recovery room. She explained we'd need to tend to the wound from the incision in the coming days, and that a visiting nurse would be arranged to assist us. We shook hands, and as she turned her back I filed her away with all the other specialists we'd seen that summer and figured we'd never see her again.

The baby we found in the recovery room resembled a corpse. He was so still, only the encouraging numbers and graphs on the bedside monitor convinced me his heart was beating and his lungs were getting oxygen. *Just wake up; just wake up*, I thought as Felicia leaned over him, praying there'd be no complications from the anesthesia.

Fifteen minutes of beeping and outside foot traffic later, the grip of his tiny hand returned as he clutched Felicia's index finger. He came to, crying in discomfort from the intubation. He was scared, pale, and miserable . . . but alive.

We made it home the following day, but the post-op routine was daunting. Sebastian was on a fresh round of antibiotics now, as the infection had been diagnosed as the *Klebsiella* bacteria. This required force-feeding him the nasty medicine. In our case, that meant holding his mouth open and placing the dropper on the back of his tongue. "That's nothin'," said Vincent, a linebacker-sized visiting nurse who looked like he could open bottles of Schlitz with his teeth as deftly as he could clean an infant's surgical wound. "I've seen parents and nurses use Hulk Hogan headlocks to make sure medicine gets swallowed on schedule." Our technique was much less forceful, but it was not the kind of loving interaction we envisioned having with our baby.

The medicine made him poop constantly, and while we had years of dirty diaper changes under our belts the situation was complicated by the need to keep the wound on his butt clean with regular applications of hydrogen peroxide. Even with Vincent's help, the Sisyphean challenge of keeping a baby's rectal area germ-free while fighting back a rising tide of excrement was a full-time job.

This went on for two weeks while he healed. The realignment of our lives to the imperatives of our baby's unanticipated health issues was depressing on the one hand but also a reinforcement of our family bonds. Marriage is, among other things, a commitment to manage big projects together as a couple, be it the wedding itself, buying a house, dealing with career challenges, or the duties of raising kids. This wasn't fun, but it was what we'd signed up for. And by now Sebastian was well into his fourth month, that stage when, still nonverbal, babies transmogrify from cooing blobs into little individuals with unique personalities, capable of genuine relationships. He'd been through so much, and yet he was eager to embrace the world, to laugh and play, to give and receive love.

Three weeks later, as the lazy days of August gave way to the hectic, hyperproductive routines of September, I was getting dressed for work when Felicia called me over to Sebastian's crib. Surprise—a second abscess had appeared in the same area, somewhat larger than the first and an angrier red.

"We're *not* putting this kid through another surgery," I hissed. "There *has* to be some other treatment option." Accordingly, I pressed Edelstein to send us to a different pediatric surgeon. I wasn't just shopping for a second opinion, I wanted a ratification of *my* opinion.

That doctor, who shall remain nameless, was obliging enough to tell me what I wanted to hear. We could try another round of antibiotics, he said, a stronger drug called clindamycin, plus a regimen of warm compresses and sitz baths. He assured me this was likely to do the trick. I left his office a satisfied customer.

After two days, it seemed the abscess was shrinking. I was so elated I convinced myself Sebastian was continuing to progress over the following days when, in fact, the abscess was expanding subcutaneously and with it, Sebastian's pain. Every time he pooped he burst out crying, his eyes shut tight as tears leaked from the edges, his smooth tongue wagging about his toothless gums as he alternately screamed and gulped for air.

My mom came for a scheduled visit and took measure of the situation. When I told her with a straight face I thought things were on the upswing she stared at me in disbelief and distrust, the same expression with which I imagined the Inca greeted Pizarro. By the weekend, I surrendered. Another surgery was the only solution.

New surgeon, new hospital, same process—but this visit to Hospitalworld distinguished itself in one important regard: it was the first time I caught a passing glimpse of horror. On the pediatric floor where we were sent post-op, I paused as I passed a patient's room crowded with visitors. Inside, a family had just received some devastating news. Within seconds relatives began pouring out of the doorway, openly sobbing and embracing each other, desperate for comfort. A despondent teenage girl who resembled a young Butterfly McQueen made eye contact with me for a second as she looked around for someone to hug. Ashamed of my intrusion, I scurried back to Sebastian's room like a busted Peeping Tom. Despite breathtaking advances in medical science, the hard truth still held: *some kids just don't make it.* For the first time I'd seen up close what that meant.

Two days later we were back home trying to manage the same postoperative procedure. The six-foot-three Vincent had befriended the four-foot-eleven Mercedes. By now I was trying to embrace the whole ordeal—the sleep deprivation, the tears, the medicine, the wound care—as a personal challenge, a test of stamina. It was therefore a staggering blow when, after ten days of meticulous care, the new wound began seeping pus and turning red at the edges. The infection had returned. We'd failed. Sebastian would need surgery yet again on the same spot.

This would have been an unassailable opportunity for Felicia to make me feel even worse, but she rose above it. We were still a team. We returned, mendicant, to Dr. Mossberg, who in her consummate professionalism suppressed what must have been a seismic urge to say "I told you so." Sebastian went under the knife for the third time on October 5.

"I've had enough of the 'some babies just get these' explanations," Felicia announced when we finally made it home. She'd come to suspect something systemic was awry with her baby. The answer, she believed, had something to do with his little body's ability to fight off infection. At her insistence, we booked an appointment with an immunologist. "This was my child, and I had to take action because no one else was," she recalled. "No one was connecting the dots."

Well, perhaps one person was. "*Sí, señora,*" agreed a nodding Mercedes when Felicia told her about the immunologist appointment. "*Buena idea.*"

Dr. Ronit Herzog began her career as a pediatric pulmonologist, but after a few years she felt the field wasn't satisfying her innate curiosity. Herzog is one of those doctors who could have been a detective, gifted with a knack for making sense out of fragmented evidence. The kind of person who focuses on the background of a painting and follows the middle voicings in orchestral music. For her the mysterious, fascinating world of immunology was a natural fit: the field is suited to those who can spot exotic conditions camouflaged behind common symptoms. How? By looking hard enough and asking the right questions.

By my reading of the medical records, Herzog was the nineteenth specialist to examine, treat, or operate on our son. Thankfully she'd familiarized herself with his medical history, so we didn't have to perform it for her. She did, however, pepper us with probing questions about what else might be troubling him. Any cough, diarrhea, breathing issues? Anyone in the family come down with an infection recently? And what about environmental factors—is he usually at home while the apartment gets dusted? Near any lawn clippings or damp areas with mold and mildew? What kind of floors do we have? And just as we thought she was through, a classic Columbo just-one-more-thing: Any pets? "In immunology we don't just do standard blood tests," she explained in an accent straight from a Tel Aviv souk. "A big part of the job is selecting the *right* tests to do." The Columbo act was simply her way of gathering investigative leads.

In Sebastian's case, medical science wasn't going to be an exact science. On the one hand, he was thriving physically. His solid position on the height and weight charts (59th and 70th percentiles, respectively) meant his body hadn't been diverting energy required for growth to fight off chronic infection. For Herzog that ruled out severe combined immunodeficiency, or SCID—the famous "boy in the bubble" condition most people of my generation know from the John Travolta biopic of David Vetter, the child who gained national attention after being born with the disease in 1971. (FYI, the SCID community considers the film anathema.)

Also, Herzog said, kids typically get an average of ten infections before they start kindergarten. Sebastian had had two, maybe three within his first five months. This could have been nothing more than an unfortunate front-loading of his normal allotment.

The red flag was that second, recurrent abscess, the one that required two surgeries. The records showed his white blood cell count was elevated at the time—clearly his body had sensed infection and dispatched the appropriate cells to fight it off. So . . . why hadn't they done their job?

The decision to start screening for an immune deficiency was a subjective call. Herzog made it without reservation. "Some people say only do the minimum tests to be cost-effective," she told me, "but my priority is to shorten the time to diagnosis. I need to know what to do."

More tests meant more blood draws. By now Sebastian's arm veins had been punctured so many times the phlebotomist needed to use his hand. The vein was tough to find. It took three attempts.

The simplest and quickest of Herzog's tests were blood count differentiations—these would determine if Sebastian's immune system was producing the proper *quantities* of cells. They came back either normal or high. Translation: his system was producing enough cellular soldiers to fight infection. That was good.

By now we were so starved for positive news we didn't bother to sift through the details. Sebastian was recovering from his third surgery in two months and we'd been bombarded with so many test results they were hard to keep straight. "His immune system is producing the proper number of cells." I took that to mean we'd eliminated any immunological issues. End of story.

Ten days later I was in my office feeling hopeful for the first time in months. At 6:30 I turned from my desk and slid some papers into my briefcase. I was reaching for my coat when my phone rang. It was Dr. Herzog's office calling, presumably to sort out some insurance matter or to schedule a routine follow-up.

"Mr. Sancho?"

"Yes, hi."

"Please hold for Dr. Herzog."

Five seconds of silence. Mercifully, no Seals & Crofts hold Muzak.

"Mr. Sancho?"

"Yes, Dr. Herzog."

"Mr. Sancho, are you sitting down?"

Chapter 3

Overboard

....

The immune system is vital. It protects the body from a constant assault of microbial attacks. You can survive a long time with an untreated, totally dysfunctional reproductive system. An untreated, totally dysfunctional immune system guarantees premature death.

The immune system is a network. It operates within and throughout the body on the cellular level, from the surface of your skin to your spit to your bones. You cannot be shot through the immune system the way you can be shot through the liver.

The immune system is a team. A diverse but disciplined army of cells, each with its own genetic composition and instructions, has evolved to beat back a shape-shifting rogues' gallery of pathogens. Viruses, bacteria, fungi—the immune system's superfriends can put forth heroes to confront millions of them.

The immune system is a student. The *innate* immune system is fixed from birth, but the *acquired* immune system (also called the *adaptive* immune system) designs customized antibodies as it encounters new attackers over time. That's why vaccinations work—the system learns and it remembers.

The immune system is a trickster. It plays games with the body, harassing other parts for no obvious reason when it gets too excited.

From this disloyalty springs the class of conditions we call autoimmune diseases: psoriasis, lupus, rheumatoid arthritis.

The immune system is a miracle. Its powers are only now beginning to be understood and harnessed. Today it is being deployed to treat various forms of cancer. Soon it may unlock the secrets of Alzheimer's disease, perhaps even clinical depression.

The immune system is a mystery. Immunology's clinical studies and experiments are grounded in hard science, but the field is also notorious for spawning abstract theories—some which might be considered philosophies—of how and why the system works the way it does.

I knew next to none of this when Dr. Herzog came on the phone. I was familiar with the basic reasons we get immunized; why diseases like polio and diphtheria have been essentially eradicated in the United States; how Pasteur, Semmelweis, and Salk earned their places in the pantheon of modern medicine. I also knew a bit about AIDS, but hadn't that been basically dealt with too?

I didn't know much because I didn't need to. I regarded my immune system the way I regarded my smartphone. It worked—that was enough. So when Dr. Herzog cleared her throat and informed me additional testing had revealed Sebastian had a primary immune deficiency called CGD, it was easy for me to reject what she said.

"Wait, *what?*" I stammered into the phone. "Something's wrong. Last week when the tests came back you told us his immune system was doing what it was supposed to."

No, she explained, her demeanor as impervious to provocation as a Buckingham Palace guard. The prior tests only confirmed his immune system was manufacturing the proper *quantities* of cells to fight infection. This one additional test—for this one rare disease—gauged the *quality* of those cells. Were they functional? Could they do their job?

The results were conclusive: no.

Herzog proceeded to remind me respectfully how she'd gone over all this weeks earlier. Ever the medical detective, she'd resolved to leave no stone unturned, no offbeat scenario unexplored. That, of course, is the immunologists' art—to look for zebras, not just horses, when they hear the sound of hooves.

The methodical approach required her to test for CGD, a peculiar condition in which one type of white blood cell, a type of granulocyte called a neutrophil, just doesn't work. "I didn't make a big deal out of it at the time," she said, "because while the first symptoms can appear common, CGD is extremely rare. It occurs in only one out of every two hundred and fifty thousand births."

I've spoken to several other parents who've received the same diagnosis and reacted with the same disbelief I did. Many tell the same story of forgetting that a test for this rare disease was ever ordered. The brain locks in on that word—*rare*—and uses it as an excuse to reject the possibility of the test coming back positive, rounding the minuscule odds down to zero. This is how winning lottery tickets go unclaimed and wind up lost in pants pockets, laundered into oblivion.

Now it all came back, and with it the news: our number had hit.

I too resisted the diagnosis. "How can you be sure this wasn't a false positive?" As I heard myself barking at the facts like a poodle at a postman, I felt an annihilating dread rising from my stomach. The walls of my office started closing in like the *Star Wars* trash compactor. My only defensive maneuver was assuming the posture of a skeptical journalist, valiantly but hopelessly straining to discredit Herzog's conclusions and restore the universe to its prior equilibrium.

Herzog was prepared for this. It's true, she acknowledged, there are a variety of factors that can yield incorrect results. Dramatic temperature changes or delays during the shipping of the sample, for instance, can make it appear the cells aren't potent, when in fact they've just been damaged from mishandling. "To make sure that hasn't happened," she said, "the patient's blood is always shipped together with a control sample from an unrelated volunteer whose blood is drawn at the same place and time. In this case I used my own."

She agreed with me that the test should be repeated and encouraged us to get a second opinion. But she was sufficiently confident in these first results to insist on seeing us immediately. If her diagnosis was correct, we needed to act. Now. We set an appointment for 9 a.m. the following morning and I hung up.

In 2003 a former army paratrooper named Tim Sears fell ten stories off one of the upper decks of the Carnival cruise ship *Celebration*. According to news reports, he lost consciousness during the fall; when he came to he found himself in the Gulf of Mexico, in the pitch-black dark, watching the distant lights from the ship's stern receding into the distance. One question dominated his thoughts: *How did I get here?*

To the degree I'm able to describe how I felt as I sat back down, Mr. Sears's story comes close. The sudden and overwhelming feelings of disorientation, of a profound loss of bearing, of mortal fear, combined with an acute awareness of one's past and future—the life our family had been living minutes before and the life we'd been expecting to lead henceforth—steaming over the horizon and out of view. In an instant, I'd been dunked into a piss-warm sea and left alone to fight off a smack of jellyfish.

I spent a few seconds listening to the hum of my office building's HVAC system. Then at some point my right arm picked up the phone again and put the receiver next to my skull. The left hand dialed Felicia. She was at home working at her desk and picked up on the second ring. "I've got something to tell you," she recalled me saying, and I'm grateful she remembered me saying it tenderly.

I have no idea how Felicia and I functioned that evening, but we managed to keep up appearances during a family dinner, story time, and lights-out. (Felicia credits a short-lived delusion that the condition could be managed through diet.) Sebastian and Lydia were sharing our small second bedroom, and as I looked in on their angelic faces before closing their door for the night, I reflected on how dismal their futures now looked. I recalled a Christmas Eve sermon I'd heard in church a few years before. "The Nativity scene is so poignant," the priest had observed, "because we know where the story goes. That baby ends up on a cross."

That night it happened for the first time. Vexed to nightmare by images of an empty cradle, I awoke at 3 a.m. to a cacophony of dark and noisy thoughts. There may be no lonelier place on earth than your own bedroom in the middle of the night with no one to talk to and no way to sleep.

Of the various white blood cells that comprise the innate immune system—the part that works automatically at birth—the neutrophil is the most abundant and among the most important first responders. When the body detects bacterial or fungal infection, neutrophils swarm to the site and proceed to eat the cells of those pathogens. In the process they release an enzyme called NADPH oxidase that, in turn, breaks down into hydrogen peroxide. That hydrogen peroxide then kills the infection.

Sebastian's neutrophils, though abundant and motile, could eat the infectious cells but could *not* produce the NADPH oxidase—there was zero "oxidative burst," to use the doctors' phrase. When he got an infection, the neutrophils would answer the call, but the pathogens would not die. This would provoke the body to produce and dispatch yet more neutrophils, which, like their progenitors, were doomed to fail. The buildup of dysfunctional neutrophils causes a nodule, called a granuloma, to form at the site of infection. A person with dysfunctional neutrophils will get these with regularity. Thus the clunky name CGD—chronic granulomatous disease.

"It mostly affects boys through the X chromosome," Herzog explained to us the next morning, a stone-faced assistant at her side. She went on to lay out her plan to conduct genetic testing to confirm the diagnosis.

With my brain befogged by sleeplessness and stress, I grasped maybe half of the immunology lecture, but that genetic thing got my attention. It aroused a hope this could all be a mistake. After all, if this were a hereditary genetic condition, wouldn't there have been some family history of it? To the best of my knowledge there was no such prior case decorating the branches of Sebastian's genealogy.

As I pondered, Herzog's colleague proceeded to bullet-point our new reality:

- The condition wasn't going away. This thing was permanent and if not managed properly, it would be fatal. The good news was that there were no current signs of infection. From this point onward, our entire lives would be an organized, continuous effort to maintain that status quo.

- That meant, for starters, a permanent prescription for prophylactic antibiotic and antifungal medications. He'd be taking multiple doses, daily, for the rest of his life. The medicines would reduce the risk of infection. They would not eliminate it.

- Therefore we had to avoid, literally like the plague, any contact with all sources of bacterial and fungal infection. The list included, but was not limited to: cut grass, mulch, hay, lakes, dirt, sand, raked leaves, sick or recently sick people.

· CGD patients are at risk of chronic inflammation as well as infection. We should expect one or more gastrointestinal issues to arise, such as Crohn's or some other inflammatory bowel disease.

· Thankfully, the part of his immune system that fights viruses was intact (neutrophils fight bacteria and fungi only), so Sebastian wouldn't have to live in a bubble. But even with the most conscientious care, they told us, we should expect him to contract a life-threatening infection once every three or four years.

"Is that the best we can hope for?" I asked.

"There is only one curative treatment," Herzog's colleague answered, pausing for a breath before she said the words, as if summoning the courage to utter the name Sauron: "a bone marrow transplant."

She went on to explain a bit about what that was—a lengthy procedure that typically involves intense chemotherapy to wipe out the existing immune system (the cells of which are manufactured in the marrow of the bones); the introduction of cells from a matched donor, assuming one can be found; and an extended, painful and risky process of recovery in which setback was a near certainty and success was not.

"The room became blurry," Felicia recalled. "The doctors' words seemed to come in slow motion. I looked around the room and thought about grabbing Sebastian and running away. Then I realized we were trapped."

One mother who got the same news about her son remembers maintaining her composure until she tried to stand up and walk out of the room. She collapsed in the hallway and wept, head in hands, knees on the sheet-vinyl flooring. When another family got its CGD diagnosis, the father asked his wife to pick up their baby from the examination table. He'd started feeling sick and had to lie down. "He'd never faced a major medical problem," his wife told me. "For someone like that, it can be overwhelming."

Felicia and I managed to hold it together, in part because Dr. Herzog made it clear the situation was urgent. His excellent presentation notwithstanding, Sebastian was very much in danger. In many cases, CGD patients have partial neutrophil function. Sebastian had zero—the most acute variation of the condition one could have. Given that, plus his history of multiple infections at such a young age (most patients aren't diagnosed till age three), it was entirely likely he'd get another one soon if we didn't act fast. And his next abscess could pop up in a hideously difficult-to-reach, life-threatening part of the body—the liver, the intestines, the lungs, the bones.

Herzog wrote the prescriptions and ordered a repeat of the tests—despite her confidence in the diagnosis, she required concrete certainty. As we rose to leave she handed us some literature on local support groups.

Trying to be strong for Felicia, I volunteered to go down the hall and handle the freshly ordered blood draw.

Edelstein the pediatrician once told me babies have a wide menu of cries, each customized for a specific message—one for "I'm hungry," one for "I'm wet," one for "I'm tired." That morning in Herzog's office the nurse failed to find a vein, not once but three times, and Sebastian's piercing screams sent an accusatory message I'd never heard before—*"What are you letting them do to me?"* His eyes shot me a look of terrified betrayal.

That's when I lost it. I stormed out of the room and pounded the wall of the hallway. "GodDAMMMMMit!" I bellowed, head bowed, tears splashing onto the inside surface of my glasses. We left without drawing the sample.

Back home, after picking up the medicines—a Pepto-Bismolish fluid called Bactrim and a syrup named itraconazole—we went through the motions of our evening routine. After the kids went down I slouched over to the house iMac and googled "chronic granulomatous disease," a colossal mistake on par with my 1999 Enron investment.

The personal testimonies were chronicles of crippling infections, Lent-long hospital stays, and miserable side effects (stunted growth, irritable bowel syndrome, acne). Seeking refuge in the antiseptic language of medical research, I pulled up some papers on PubMed. Coiled among the bricks of tiny text, one fanged and venomous statistic sprang out—"Average life expectancy for CGD patients is approximately thirty years."

Heart pounding, head throbbing, I stood up from the desk and lumbered to bed. Slithering under the covers, I turned to Felicia for a cuddle, hoping she was asleep. Instead she was silently sobbing. I ran my fingers through her long brown hair, already anticipating how this calamity was going to disfigure our lives as a couple. Her thoughts were elsewhere. "I'm just thinking of Lydia. What this is going to mean for *her*." I had no answers, and I didn't want to share the headlines from my online research. We whimpered ourselves to sleep.

The next morning I was a zombie at work. For the first time in my life I'd been confronted with an unsolvable, unignorable problem. Forget about the auto-shop attitude toward medicine. This time there was no simple repair. This could not be fixed. All my life I'd been the kid with the magnifying glass; now I was the ant.

The afternoon senior staff meeting was an opportunity to test my powers of compartmentalization; to block out the nightmare by attending to professional responsibilities—story selection, scheduling, staffing, budgets. An hour and a half later, as the meeting wound down and small talk began its conquest of the conversation, a colleague asked after Sebastian. The group had all been immensely supportive during the chaos of the past months, and I figured this was a good time to break the news, so I asked for the room's attention and laid out the facts quickly.

I consider business attire armor more than clothing, and I was counting on my gray suit, tie, and cuff links to provide adequate fortification against breaking down in front of my boss. I counted wrong—all my defenses collapsed, the levee broke. I was a blubbering mess.

That same afternoon Felicia was back at Herzog's office for the second attempt at the blood draw. A Haitian technician was on duty, and she executed the task with breathtaking ease. After checking in with the doctors, Felicia headed to the elevator and bumped into her again. Her name was Theresa, and to Felicia's surprise she suddenly dropped her façade of professionalism and leaned in for a hug.

"I felt safe in her presence," Felicia recounted, "and I began to cry. Deep and heavy sobs from the pit of my stomach. When we finally pulled apart, she held my shoulders, looked straight in my eyes, and said with conviction, 'Don't give up on him. He is going to prove the doctors wrong. You will see.'"

Then she began to pray. After a big "Amen," she made the following guarantee:

"He's going to be okay," she said, almost defiantly. "You will see."

"How can you be so sure?" Felicia responded.

"Because anything is possible with faith," she said.

This was one of several numinous encounters that would punctuate Felicia's life for the next six years, chance run-ins with angels through whom she found inspiration and strength for the journey. The theologian John Dominic Crossan compares God to a courtesy outlet in an airport—a source of replenishing energy for the smartphone of your soul, there for free for you to access, whether or not you know you need it. Felicia has always been prepared to plug in. That openness has served her well.

I, however, could not join her. Even in my most spiritual moods, I could never conceive of the divine operating on the cellular level. That was the realm of science, and it was in these doctors I resolved to entrust my faith. For my own sustenance, I opted for steely stoicism. After the emasculating nature of the Hospitalworld experience and the embarrassment of my public crying, I wanted nothing more than to emulate the noble, battle-scarred survivors I'd been putting on TV for years—parents who'd lost kids in plane crashes, wars, and abductions and yet found the strength to assimilate their tragedy, tell their stories, and move forward. Hardship was a part of life; I was a grown man and I'd just learn to handle it.

My birthday was the following weekend and Felicia had crammed it with enough activity to crowd out some of the misery. We went back to the Catskills and stayed at a lodge adjacent to the Bear Mountain Oktoberfest. The event gets savaged on Yelp for the obscene lines at the brat house and beer tents, but for us it was a joyous relief just to be out of a medical environment doing something with regular people.

On the drive home, we made a pit stop along one of the river towns for a snack and a diaper change. It was Felicia's turn and she attended to Sebastian in the back seat while I took a brief stroll with Lydia. When I returned, my wife's beautiful brown eyes, always large, had swollen into kalamata olives.

"Sebastian's wound. It's reinfected."

I looked. She was right. The abscess area was a nasty purple; yellow pus was seeping out.

We didn't flinch. Felicia, in fact, was relieved—in light of the diagnosis, this all made sense for once. And she knew the drill—call doctor, pack overnight bag, eat something, head to hospital, find a phlebotomist with pediatric specialty to prevent a bad blood draw.

The underreaction was warranted. This time Sebastian wouldn't need surgery. Dr. Mossberg managed to clean out the wound and sent him home with a prescription for yet another, stronger antibiotic. I was in the apartment with Lydia when Felicia called with the news. I put her to bed and, stroking her forehead after she slept, looked forward to a time when Sebastian's health had stabilized. If only this one lingering infection would clear, if only we could get out of capital *C* crisis mode, then we could start strategizing for the long term. We just needed a respite between the volleys of slings and arrows.

After ripping through Jamaica, Cuba, and the Bahamas, Superstorm Sandy turned north toward the United States on Saturday, October 27. In New York a deluge of apocalyptic warnings had already begun. The *New York Post*, ever creative, reworked an image of Boris Karloff to make its "Frankenstorm" cover.

I was skeptical. Personally familiar with how news outlets hype weather events, I suspected this would turn out to be another meteorological dud. Plus, compared to what we'd already endured, nature's fury was a source of mirth. We didn't even bother to check the batteries in our flashlights.

Five hours later, the storm surge inundated Battery Park. NYU Langone Hospital was evacuated after flooding knocked out its generators. The lights were going out in lower Manhattan. It occurred to me that if the blackout spread above 49th Street, we'd have no way to keep Sebastian's medicine refrigerated, no reliable means of transportation, and perhaps no hospital to take him to if his condition worsened. Plus, who knows what infectious disease outbreaks might emerge from the bowels of a flooded city with no power. This was not what we needed.

"Is it just me," Felicia remarked, "or does it feel like the world is ending?"

Chapter 4

PWASK

....

On the third day, the waters receded.

The blackout stayed below 34th Street; our lights stayed on. Outside, emergency service crews nursed the city's infrastructure back to life; inside, we nursed our son back to health. Outside, the storm prompted many to ponder the fickle moods of the planet and its climate; inside, our family's attentions were glued to the goings-on at the cellular level inside Sebastian's body. The rest of the world could look at life through a wide-angle lens; from now on we'd be viewing it through a microscope.

Sebastian had stabilized, his wound was healing, the prophylactic regimen of medicines seemed to be protecting him. Had Tom Ridge been changing my son's diapers, he would have lowered the threat alert from red to yellow. On Halloween we trick-or-treated, Manhattan style, among the apartments in our building; Lydia was Madeline, Sebastian a strawberry in a stroller. If you squinted a bit, we looked like a normal family.

With Sebastian's storm quieted and our diagnostic odyssey concluded, our next big step was going public. Felicia and I had been hesitant to tell people because, as I'd discovered when I broke the news to my closest colleagues, it was nearly impossible to speak the necessary words without weeping. It takes energy and time to recover from those hemorrhages of emotion; we didn't have the stamina to repeat that agonizing exercise ad nauseam.

I even delayed telling my family because, out in California, my sister had given birth to a baby girl the same week as Sebastian's diagnosis. My mother had made the trip west for the occasion. I didn't want to "yuck their yum," much less strike the fear of congenital disease into my sister's postpartum brain, awash with hormones. When I finally made the call, I choked back the tears and kept it short.

Forgoing any further one-on-one conversations, we opted for a group email, despite the imperfections of the medium. After a few drafts, I thought I'd struck the proper balance of sober reportage and acknowledgment of our fears and frailty. The conclusion went heavy on hope. Knowing this email would permanently alter how our friends perceived us, I took a deep breath and hit send.

It's tough to convey sympathy in an email reply without stomping on at least one of the twin land mines of callousness and cliché. The messages that hit our in-boxes in the following minutes reflected the same struggle, and I felt bad for obliging my closest friends to compose them.

Amid the If-there's-anything-we-can-dos and the he's-got-two-of-the-world's-best-parentses, there were a few inevitable smatterings of the reliable platitude—"God never gives you more than you can handle"—a coin so widely circulated in our culture its face has worn off. "We'll see about that," I muttered to myself. At least we were spared that old chestnut "Everything happens for a reason."

It's not that I resented my friends' support. To clarify: I resented the fact that I *needed* my friends, support. Misfortune can be a designator of social status as much as ethnicity, class, or education. Parents with a sick kid—PWASK as we came to refer to ourselves—are in their own caste—the quintessential members of a club no one wants to join. Pity is a soft form of cruelty, and the thought that our family was now to be

a designated charity case made my stomach turn. Another rare disease dad I'd meet later said it best: "I didn't want people to look at us
weird. I didn't want us to be known as the family with *that kid.*" As the
sympathetic replies kept hitting my in-box, my soul sprang a leak.
Over time the seepage would become a deep pool of bitterness. I had
always been loath to identify with the classic victim mentality—the
surrender to powerlessness, the belief that one's life is controlled by
large unseen forces, the fixation on problems. And yet that identity
was threatening to engulf us.

That's why I threw out the support group brochures Dr. Herzog had
handed us, and why we posted nothing publicly about the diagnosis on
Facebook. It was bad enough our closest friends had to see this ugly
new scar on our faces. We saw no need to let it redefine the attenuated
relationships we maintained online. As any user knows, social media
is an oppressive onslaught of tailored happiness; any bad news lands
like a turd in a punch bowl. So long as Sebastian provided a steady
stream of cute baby pics to upload, we could keep his condition semi-
secret and maintain a Facebook fiction that all was well.

This launched an unplanned social experiment—observing the behavior of the friends we hadn't told (the control group) against those we
had. The control group continued with its occasional hey-theres and
let's-get-togethers. The experimental group split into two cohorts—
those who gravitated closer to us and those who drifted away.

I'm infinitely grateful we had a wealth of support from those who
stepped up, offered to help, or simply checked in. Just knowing they
were there made a tremendous difference. As for those who distanced
themselves—who can really blame them? The demands of work and
family are so immense, few people have the time or emotional capacity
to take on someone else's problems.

Then there's that other thing, the thing nobody talks about—the
superstitious feeling that bad fortune is contagious. At least in the

success cult that is New York City, setback is synonymous with failure, and failure is to be avoided like the Port Authority Bus Terminal after the bars close on St. Patrick's Day.

It's common for the PWASK to grow isolated from their friends and even their own families. A CGD mom from an unnamed Southern state told me that when she informed her family about her son's diagnosis, they were in the middle of a character breakfast at Disney World. Their immediate concern, she said, was for themselves. A sibling: "Oh my God, could this happen to *my* kids?" A parent: "I hope you're not blaming *me* for this." After a round of perfunctory condolences, they took some photos with Lilo and Stitch and proceeded with their scheduled vacation. "I tried to explain the genetics of it to them, but they couldn't wrap their brains around it," she told me. "They wanted to make sure they couldn't 'catch it,' which of course is impossible with a genetic condition. And they really didn't want my sad all over them." Many of her friends reacted similarly. "I didn't want pity, I just wanted love. I wanted people to come together. But they just wanted to go about their lives. They didn't really understand or want to understand. They didn't grasp the severity of it at all."

For families of the immunodeficient, that social alienation is compounded by self-imposed physical isolation. Fighting a war without guns against microscopic enemies, one's instinct is to retreat into a defensive crouch. Starting on the day of the diagnosis, Felicia and I began ascending an Everest of germophobia. We enforced a strict no-shoes policy at home. We obsessively Lysol-wiped every surface we touched; our Purell budget mushroomed. And we dialed all discretionary human contact way back—hand shaking, out; playdates with other kids, strictly verboten pending further notice. Long before "social distancing" became a household term, it was our household norm. In short, we turtled up.

* * *

Weeks passed. Things happened. We barely noticed it, but there was a presidential election and Barack Obama won a second term.

Felicia and I assured ourselves we could adapt to this new life and make it work—others certainly had—but emotionally we were living in a house of straw, and the lightest breeze could blow it down.

A certified letter arrived in mid-November—the results of the DNA testing Dr. Herzog had ordered. Her hypothesis that Sebastian's CGD was linked to his X chromosome was confirmed. No surprise there, but the news landed on Felicia like an anvil. One thing we knew for sure—Sebastian had received his Y chromosome from his father, this bad X from his mom. After reading the results identifying a monogenetic mutation on the CYBB gene on that same X—she collapsed. In her mind, she'd condemned her own son to a life of suffering.

"A *mutation*!" she sobbed, fetal-positioned on the couch. "I'm a *mutant*! A malformed human being! I always wanted to be a mother, but I should *never* have had kids!" Aside from Sebastian's predicament, she was also lamenting the 50 percent chance that Lydia was a carrier (we hadn't tested her, so we didn't know). If Lydia had the bad X, my X would prevent her from having CGD, but she could pass it on to *her* male kids. Like other CGD moms I've spoken to, Felicia read the DNA results as a personal indictment. "You feel labeled, you feel damaged," one mom told me. "I unknowingly passed this horrible disease on to my children. And it has broken me completely."

"I've always felt that somehow I was not good enough," Felicia admitted that night. "It was a deep, hidden sense of doom. Now I have proof."

I said what I was supposed to say as I rubbed her back. "Don't beat yourself up. It's not your fault. There've been no prior cases in your family; there was no way we could have known." I meant every word, but I felt like a bad actor.

Felicia got up to turn off the living room lights. Then she sat back down on the couch and continued to cry in the dark. She said she wanted to be alone.

Later as I lay in our bed, staring at the ceiling as the sound of her meek sniffles came through the door, my stoicism foundered. I put my head under a pillow and screamed at the top of my lungs. (Years later, I'd read that this was a therapeutically valid anger management technique.) *"I HATE . . . THIS FUCKING . . . DISEASE!"*

I hated what it was doing to my wife.

I hated what I could foresee it doing to my daughter, my marriage, my finances.

I hated how it made some people look at my son.

I hated how it was forcing me to recalibrate my life's goals and expectations.

I hated the human body.

I hated the world.

I hated God.

The next morning I awoke from a dreamless sleep and remembered something that had happened days before at the office. A colleague who'd just learned of Sebastian's condition had entered my office, come around my desk, put his hands on my shoulders, and given me some of the clearest, best advice I've ever received: "Don't think about the big picture. That will overwhelm you. Just deal with what's right in front of you." Bearing that simple wisdom in mind, I arose and just dealt with what was in front of me—giving Sebastian that morning's medicine.

The holidays rolled around and we were suddenly taking them quite seriously. We didn't discuss it much, but Felicia and I knew Sebastian's first Thanksgiving and Christmas could also be his last. My parents had divorced years ago and my mom now lived in Philly. We went to her house and tried to enjoy some quiet, sacred togetherness, focusing intently on the meaning and spirit of gratitude.

Unfortunately, even while we were singing "'Tis a Gift to Be Simple" around my mom's rickety piano, part of us was decaying. A long-term psychological erosion had begun, which I didn't comprehend until it was explained to me years later, by Dr. Amy Arnsten, a professor of neuroscience at Yale School of Medicine. Professor Arnsten studies the effects of stress on the brain, particularly the prefrontal cortex, where much of human higher cognitive functioning takes place.

"For the PFC to work at its optimum capacity," she told me, "its brain cells have to excite each other through the circuits of the synapses." In periods of stress, a subset of neurons right next to the synapses gets activated and special chemical pathways called potassium channels open. This inhibits the ability of those brain cells to communicate through the synapses. The circuits grow silent, inhibiting crucial functions like abstract reasoning, planning, and language, as well as important stamina and confidence boosters like the ability to be one's own best cheerleader.

Conversely, the more primitive parts of the brain, the amygdala especially, hyperactivate. This region controls emotional responses and associations. Stress floods these regions with norepinephrine and dopamine, amping up our sensory perception. Cortisol, released by the adrenal cortex, blocks the reuptake of those chemicals, reinforcing the effect.

From an evolutionary perspective, this makes sense. When confronted with a life-and-death situation it's more advantageous to have the contemplative part of the brain take a back seat to the reactive region governing the fight-or-flight response. Strategizing, insight, and compassion for your partner can be put on hold. That's what spawned

49

today's medical consensus that acute stress is a good, necessary thing for survival—the nervous system has a way to handle physical threats, just as the immune system has its ways to handle infectious disease.

Chronic stress is another story. "The chronic stress studies in rodents indicate two things happening," Dr. Arnsten explained. "The chemical pathways opened by acute stress get stronger over time, to the point that you have changes in the physical architecture of the brain. In the prefrontal cortex, the dendrites within the brain cell body (the trees and spines) begin to atrophy. The spines start to disappear. The brain cell *is actually shrinking*."

Again, there may be an evolutionary reason for this. The prefrontal cortex consumes a sizable amount of glucose. In a chronic, ongoing crisis like a drought, it may well be advantageous for *Homo sapiens* to shut down that gas-guzzling section of our brains.

For Felicia and me, what had dried up and disappeared wasn't a physical resource like water but a psychological resource—optimism. The decision to have kids is inherently a vote of confidence in the future, but one's perspective shifts after you're told you're the one in the one in 250,000 whose kid is afflicted with a rare disease. It becomes very hard to believe that you won't *always* be on the losing end of long odds. The whole world dims.

For Felicia, that negativity continued to feed her secret anxieties and insecurities, striking at her confidence as a person and a woman.

She also worried that she had done something wrong while pregnant, although the doctors assured her that was not the case.

"I feel so guilty," she told me one night after the kids were asleep. "I can't stop thinking that I caused this. When I hold Sebastian and look at his perfect, beautiful face, I feel so much love and so much pain and self-loathing at the same time."

"It's a genetic mutation," I assured her again. "There's nothing you could have done to cause it or prevent it." Still, she could not shake this feeling that it was her fault, that something had always been wrong with her body. (Years later we would learn that, indeed, CGD carriers do often suffer from a variety of physical issues that go undiagnosed—including severe anxiety, skin issues, and joint pain. But the relief of that revelation was still a long way off. For now, Felicia just felt physically inferior.)

For me, chronic stress was progressively becoming my life's silent master, pulling my chains in a manner alternately gentle and violent, subtle and obvious, chewing away at my determination to remain stoic and strong.

The first sign was a creeping insomnia. "Your brain had determined that you and your loved ones were not safe," Dr. Arnsten explained years later. "It was activating low-affinity alpha-1 and beta-receptors that cause wakefulness in the thalamus." The upshot: I was lucky to get four hours of sleep per night.

A recent study shows that during non-REM sleep, waves of cerebrospinal fluid wash over the brain, scrubbing out toxins. When that doesn't happen, the buildup of metabolic by-products can lead in the long term to neurodegenerative disease like Alzheimer's.

In my case there were short-term effects too. As I amassed a sleep debt big enough to rival balance sheets at the National Bank of Greece, I grew scatterbrained. The first cracks appeared at work. One of my shows that fall aired with a factual error, a blunder actionable enough to require an on-air retraction. It wasn't all my fault, but I bore enough responsibility that some of my friends felt the need to play the "he's been having health problems with his baby" card with upper management to keep me out of serious trouble.

I knew I needed to do something to take the edge off, and my first attempt at self-help could not have been more stereotypical—self-medication with my preferred intoxicants.

Ever since age fifteen, I'd been a firm believer in the Dionysian impulse. The ability to get wasted and bust loose without regretting it terribly the next day ranked right up there with athletic or intellectual achievement.

Concerning marijuana, I was a borderline evangelist. Some of the most transcendent, creative, and loving moments of my life had been aided and abetted by cannabinoids. I considered toking an inalienable right, even after a dear friend (and an esteemed medical professional) and I had been arrested for sparking up a bowl on the Bowery.

Booze, a mini-vacation in a bottle, had become a steadfast ally as I'd aged. Gone were the days of vomiting on my shoes or waking up on the pavement, both of which I'd done in my midtwenties. By forty I'd learned to enjoy and handle liquor like a seasoned pro. Trouble was, drinking somehow made my insomnia worse. The alcohol helped me go down, but it made it harder to *stay* down. I'd pop up in bed even earlier than normal, still buzzing, with nothing but *The Economist* as a soporific.

After spending much of that Christmas season in some state of inebriation, I concluded substance abuse was an impractical long-term solution. We all want to put some distance between ourselves and reality, but escapism is fundamentally a childish endeavor. And my new responsibilities as a PWASK made it impossible to act like a child for very long. Millions of dads cut and run when things get choppy, many before their babies are even born. I was not going to be one of them, so I dialed back the bourbon and bong hits and . . . dealt with what was in front of me.

The road ahead of us stretched far beyond the horizon. We were still just getting our heads around the dimensions of our problem and how we might deal with it. Given the dearth of reliable medical advice, our immunologist Dr. Herzog said we should consult one of the handful of experts who spent their careers studying CGD.

Those referrals all pointed in the same direction—the National Institutes of Health in Bethesda, Maryland. There at NIH, the research hospital of last resort for exotic illnesses, the world's preeminent CGD expert was fighting a lifelong battle against this disease so few knew or cared about. His name was Dr. Harry Malech, and he agreed to see us the first week in January.

Felicia and I spent the last night of our *annus horribilis* on our aging Macy's couch, undrunk, watching Ryan Seacrest host *New Year's Rockin' Eve*. Times Square was one mile due west from where we were sitting. It felt a thousand light-years away.

The ball dropped.

Happy New Year.

Chapter 5

Off to See the Wizard

If architecture is frozen music, then the NIH could be Holst's "Mars, the Bringer of War." The place is staffed with superb, caring professionals, but stepping foot onto the property is tougher than boarding an El Al flight to Tel Aviv. The sprawling campus, comprised of more than seventy-five buildings, sits on three hundred acres of rolling Bethesda suburb. Before 9/11, local dog walkers and picnickers strolled the grounds unhindered. After the Pentagon was hit and the Twin Towers came down, the wrought-iron fencing went up. Today, visitors undergo the standard battery of federal security precautions, plus some extra biosecurity measures—the facility has a storied history working with infectious and toxic agents like anthrax and smallpox.

We drove up to the Gateway Inspection Station and got the full Crichton novel treatment. A somber parade through the metal detector, the scanning of our valid government IDs, a litany of repetitive questions, low-res photos of us sporting strained smiles for the visitors' passes. The security team opened and inspected all the bags in the trunk, examined every bottle of medicine and formula. A neurotic bomb-sniffing dog circumambulated our rented Town & Country twice as we stood by. Forty-five minutes after we'd arrived, a guard raised a beefy hand from the stock of his rifle and waved us through. "I feel like we've walked into the last reel of *E.T.*," Felicia muttered to me. She fought back tears as she imagined handing our baby over to feds in hazmat suits for a lifetime of experimental procedures. This was not your average doctor's visit.

After parking on some sublevel and pushing the stroller through a rat maze of passageways, we found our first friendly face. By pure coincidence, my cousin by marriage Lee England worked at the NIH and knew Dr. Malech, the wizard we'd come to see. Endowed with an otherworldly calm, she welcomed us at the admissions office and explained that, while the place is physically imposing, the people who work there are as kind and accessible as they are brilliant.

The NIH houses twenty-seven institutes and centers, each focused on its own field of research. Dr. Malech's office was part of the National Institute of Allergy and Infectious Diseases, which later shot to fame in the COVID-19 crisis. A ten-minute walk from admissions brought us to a modest, utilitarian space—the centerpiece of the waiting area was a watercooler and a small fridge with juice boxes and sodas. A large, shopworn Purell dispenser hung on the wall.

Malech met us in an exam room and I took a moment to take the measure of the man we were asking to save our son. His presentation: avuncular, a graying James Garnerish face framed by large glasses that said scientist more than physician. Cheeks that had spent approximately ten thousand times as many hours in a lab than on a beach. Curious, sad eyes that had already seen too much, yet wanted to see more.

Malech began his career in oncology but shifted to infectious disease for two reasons, one intellectual, one emotional. As a researcher, he'd become fascinated with our favorite cell, the neutrophil. "I was interested in cell movement and one of my mentors showed me how much more neutrophils move than cancer cells," he said. "They are the sprinters of the human body. The way they race to the site of infection is breathtaking."

The emotional pull was easier to grasp—at the start of his career, oncologists were losing patients more often than infectious disease specialists. Malech wanted more opportunities to save lives. "Back then, you couldn't find many patients with advanced cases of cancer and heal them," he said. "At least with infectious diseases you had a chance."

After decades in the field, Malech had likely examined more CGD patients than anyone else on the planet. Many arrived in truly frightful shape—one kid showed up at NIH with a fungal infection eating through his spine; another had an infection that had invaded the pericardium (the membrane enclosing the heart) and ruptured through the sternum. Wes Craven stuff. "We are the place of last resort," he told me. "People come here because they know we won't turn anyone down. We aren't a private hospital that has to maintain an impressive success rate to attract patients. We are not afraid to treat you . . . even if it means you could die."

Compared to the hardest cases, Sebastian's issues were a hangnail. After a required weigh-in, Malech examined him carefully and quietly. The doctor checked out the wounds on Sebastian's bottom, found them unalarming, then proceeded to review the medical records. He explained that Sebastian's history, which had been such a head-scratcher for so many other doctors, was textbook CGD. I took his ho-hum demeanor as a great sign—at last, we'd found a doctor who'd been there and done that, not once but hundreds of times.

Our New York immunologist, Dr. Herzog, had sent down the results of a prior CAT scan. Curious, I peered over Dr. Malech's shoulder as he scrolled the cross-section images, moving from the top of Sebastian's cranium down to his tarsus—not the kind of baby pictures you send to Shutterfly but adorable in a way perhaps only a parent can appreciate. The crucial areas were the thorax and abdomen, the inner organs where CGD wreaks havoc most often. Thankfully the lungs, heart, stomach, spleen, liver, and intestines all checked out. The slides of the bladder made an impression—at that cross section of the body it dominates the image—just a big empty sac nested among the bones of the pelvis, surrounded by a thin layer of flesh. "Amazing how much space it takes up, isn't it?" Malech remarked with a grin. Doctor humor.

We adjourned to a large conference room, where Malech, joined by other members of his staff, began the download. For the next three hours, while Sebastian snoozed in a bouncy seat and Lydia went on a field trip with Lee, we heard everything we ever wanted to hear about CGD, and then some. Hungry to impress the team as a knowledgeable and responsible dad—an intellectual equal, not just a charity case—I'd come with a list of questions, scrawled in a reporter's notebook. Malech recalls me trying to appear "large and in charge." Pathetic, but true.

"Parents coming with young patients have often heard only the scare stories," he said. "The available medical literature is full of problems but not solutions. My first task is to separate the facts from the myths.

"You don't need to wrap your child in Bubble Wrap and keep him indoors," he assured us. "He can get immunized. With treatment, life can be pretty normal. On the other hand, there are quite a few innocuous activities that can lead to fatal infections, and you need to be aware of those." He proceeded to enumerate the threats. Many we knew already—mulch, hay, cut grass. Others were new, unpleasant surprises—mosquito bites, construction sites, Christmas trees. I inquired wishfully whether there might be some compensatory upside to the condition, like the savant abilities some autistic kids have. "I'm afraid it doesn't work that way," Malech replied. There would be no secret superpowers, no silver linings. As long as he had this condition, the healthiest Sebastian could ever be was a strange status Malech called "not sick but not well."

Then things got more abstract. Malech laid out one of the central impediments to studying rare diseases: there are simply not many cases to study. In an era of *big* data, Malech's work suffers from the problem of *small* data. A comparison: when the Surgeon General's 1964 *Reports on Smoking and Cancer* was released, its advisory committee had reviewed seven thousand articles and dozens of large-scale, long-term studies. There was an overabundance of smokers and lung cancer patients from which to harvest data. The biggest prospective therapeutic CGD study to date had only 128 patients. The law of large numbers did not apply.

This meant very few statements about the disease could be uttered without a freight train of qualifiers and disclaimers in tow. Unknowns far outnumbered the knowns. And because the condition is so rare, its patients must contend with the usual disadvantages of living with an orphan disease—few qualified experts, fewer options for treatment, little market demand for a cure. In the history of the pharmaceutical industry, only four hundred medicines have been developed to treat seven thousand orphan diseases.

If there was any good news, it was that the paucity of clinical data meant those same qualifiers and disclaimers also applied to the scariest statistics about the disease, especially those regarding reduced life expectancy. The reported outcomes included patients born decades ago, when CGD research and immunology itself were in their own respective states of infancy. So much had happened since—and was continuing to happen—that the diagnosis was no longer considered what it used to be: a death sentence. (Indeed, when it was first identified in 1950 the condition was termed fatal granulomatous disease of childhood, since so few patients made it past ten years old.)

The first game changer in treatment had been the development of a new family of oral antifungal medications called triazoles, which reduced infection rates across the board. The first of these was introduced in the eighties, but the key breakthrough was voriconazole, patented in 1990. This was the first treatment that enabled CGD patients to recover from traditionally lethal fungal infections like aspergillosis and candidiasis. A true lifesaver.

The second leap forward was the 1999 FDA approval of a strange drug called Actimmune, which works through a protein called interferon gamma. While it does not replace or repair dysfunctional neutrophils, Actimmune somehow keeps the immune system in a permanent state of high alert, reducing the risk of infection.

Here's what makes the drug strange, Malech explained: in the one big study that measured its effects, only a small subset of Actimmune patients showed significant improved immune activity *on the cellular level*. For most patients, the drug wasn't doing what it was hoped it would do. Yet a much larger number of patients had impressive results *on the clinical level*—for some unknown reason, they didn't get sick as often. The drug *was* doing what it was hoped it would do.

How could a drug be working and *not* working at the same time? *The immune system is a mystery.* "Even to this day," Malech says, "we don't know why it's helping people. The results of that study made a lot of people uncomfortable, but I still believe in it. That's the best solid science we have."

Actimmune has its downsides—it must be given as an injection, it's expensive, and it has a handful of common unpleasant side effects, including fever, chills, muscle pain, and vivid nightmares. But the point stands: if you want to make a go of living with CGD, that option is now on the table—and patients are living longer. "Have you ever had a CGD patient who died of natural causes *unrelated* to the condition?" I asked. Malech paused and said yes. The yes was encouraging, the pause less so.

The third big development, Malech continued, has been the development of a truly curative treatment—bone marrow transplantation.

Bone marrow is the soft, spongy tissue found inside the larger bones of the body, and it is where blood cells—including all the cells of the immune system—are produced. The mere ability to conceive of transplanting bone marrow, much less accomplishing the feat, is a testament to the imaginative powers of the human species. We're not just talking about taking an organ—a kidney, say—from one body and moving it to another. We're talking about wiping out the entirety of a complex, vital system in the body and *regrowing* a new one, from scratch, with foreign cells from a donor.

This is possible, Malech explained, thanks to the magic of stem cells—the source from which every type of blood cell, red and white, is formed. These blood-forming, or hematopoietic, stem cells, residing primarily in the bone marrow, spontaneously spawn every soldier in the immune system's diverse army. The truly amazing thing is this: if you infuse the right type and quantity of donor stem cells into a patient's veins, they will somehow know just where to go and precisely what to do, reproducing the donor's immune system in the patient essentially on their own. Presto!

Three onerous criteria stand in the way of successful transplantation. First, as stated above, the patient's existing immune system and stem cells must be eliminated. This typically requires a degree of chemotherapy that can easily be fatal itself. Second, the donor cells must properly match the patient's, or they won't engraft in the donor's bones and start reproducing. Finding that match can be harder than finding a loyal spouse on Tinder. Third, you've got to keep the patient alive long enough for the new immune system to get up and running, a period of months or even years during which any infection—whether caused by the common cold or a rusty nail—is potentially fatal.

It took decades to achieve anything resembling success. The first bone marrow transplant trials, conducted in the late 1950s, had such abysmal fatality rates that the procedure would be outlawed were they conducted under today's ethical standards for research on human subjects. A seminal study published in 1977 tracked 110 transplant patients and showed only a 16 percent long-term survival rate. The first successful transplant from an unrelated donor (siblings are easier to match, identical twins automatic) didn't take place in the United States until 1979, and that patient died two years later when her leukemia came back. David Vetter, the original "boy in the bubble," had a transplant in 1983. He died from lymphoma caused by the Epstein-Barr virus four months later.

And yet, precisely because the approach was considered so radical and experimental, it has attracted a constant stream of adventurous medical scientists eager to push past the limits of current knowledge, to take on the challenge of curing the incurable, even if it means risking patients' lives. They are a breed apart—they are the transplanters* some of the most innovative and daring scientists on earth.

The grail they seek is a technique that optimizes the transplanters' holy trinity—low levels of chemotherapy, high rates of engraftment, low rates of post-engraftment complication. This quest for the perfect protocol has been going on for decades, across continents, and through the sacrifices of the patients who didn't make it. Progress has been fruitful but painful. "I think about my patients often," said Malech. "I've never forgotten a single one, and I still grieve for the ones I've lost."

Over the years as the science inched forward, a variety of techniques blossomed, survival rates increased, and transplant eventually emerged as a curative treatment for more diseases, including CGD. Malech and his colleagues at the NIH were the first in the United

---

* "Transplanter" is an informal term. Doctors who perform hematopoietic stem cell transplants are typically specialists in immunology, hematology, and/or oncology. Some might bristle at the use of the slang, but it is common in the field and employed here with maximum respect.

States to establish a transplant protocol for CGD patients, and as they began to see success, even in seriously ill patients, other centers around the country followed suit. Overall success rates are now high enough that many experts recommend transplant for young kids with the most serious type of CGD—like Sebastian.

As brilliant and kind a man as Malech is, it's easier to get straightforward advice from the Delphic oracle. Part of his maddeningly elliptical manner, he said, has to do with professional constraints. He sees it as his job to lay out options, not make the big calls. We pressed him numerous times for direct guidance on what we should do—transplant? Actimmune? Radical lifestyle changes? Each time he parried the question, primarily by reassuring us that the present moment, in which our lives were still reverberating from the initial shock of the diagnosis, was without question the worst time to commit to one course of action or another. Sebastian was being treated—we now knew what was going on, what to look for, how to mitigate risk. We had time, he assured us, to investigate various options and think things through as a family. We didn't need a decision—we needed a plan.

I flashed back to a nugget of Solomonic wisdom my father had passed down in 1983 while I was trying to navigate a teenage crush: "When in doubt," he decreed, "gather data."

We concluded our meeting with Malech on an up note. With a sheaf of consent forms signed and approved, Sebastian was now officially a patient at NIH. He could be treated there, anytime, for free, and the government would reimburse our travel expenses. This was to our tremendous benefit, but the deal wasn't something for nothing. The rarer the condition, the more valuable each new patient is for research purposes. For an immunology researcher, finding a young, freshly diagnosed CGD patient is akin to a marine biologist netting a giant squid. From here on out, our son wasn't just a sick kid: he was to be an object of study.

"We have an opportunity and a responsibility to develop large co-horts of patients with rare diseases," Malech told me. "That enables us to observe uncommon presentations, to define the range of the phe-notype, as well as the range of responses to the standard of care. More than any other facility in the world, we are able to see the bigger picture."

Before we left, Malech gave us one quirky tip. He suggested we pur-chase a bottle of something called Dakin's solution and apply it topi-cally whenever Sebastian had a break in the skin. Any such injury, even something as minor as a paper cut, was an infection risk. The solution, little more than diluted bleach, had been developed by the eponymous Dr. Henry Dakin during World War I, when the gruesome innovations of modern warfare spurred equally momentous innova-tions in wound care. Years before the discovery of penicillin, Dakin had learned, through trial and error, that this solution was the least toxic means of disinfecting the horrific injuries of trench warfare. During a conflict in which disease and wound infection posed as grave a threat to survival as machine guns and mustard gas, Dakin likely saved thousands of lives.

The irony merited a chuckle. We'd made our pilgrimage to the mecca of cutting-edge medicine only to be prescribed a hundred-year-old over-the-counter remedy. But, hey, whatever works. "Some oldies but goodies are still good for what they're good for," Malech told me, chan-neling Yogi Berra.

We left and headed to Lee's house for a family get-together. Despite my anemic efforts at maintaining relationships with my extended D.C.-area family, here they were—enough to fill a house—turning up for me and a baby they'd never met with love and support, gifts I'd done little to earn.

"There's a lesson here," said Felicia as we departed. "Family *is* wealth."

Two weeks later, back in New York, we baptized our baby. In the commotion of his first nine months, we'd given little thought to maintaining religious observance, much less hosting a formal church event. Our ability to plan and pull off a baptism was itself a sign things had steadied. In keeping with Catholic tradition, we dressed Sebastian in a white gown with a little cap, symbols of new creation. *"Mira como tu sales, mi amor,"* cooed Mercedes as she prepped him for departure. *"Eres un angelito muy hermoso!"*

Neither I nor most of our assembled guests knew much about the rituals with the oils and the candle, but our priest was kind enough to explain. Anyway, the purpose of the prayers was self-evident—blessing and protecting this sacred, fragile child. He handled all the fuss and attention like a champ.

I was skeptical anything said or done at this ceremony was going to make much difference. But it didn't matter. The community surrounding us was its own higher power. In that room, together, three dozen friends, colleagues, and family members had gathered, each committed to saving Sebastian's life. We had years of struggle ahead of us and an ocean of pain to swim across, but we would not be alone.

Chapter 6

Zugzwang

....

In a run-down storefront in downtown New Rochelle, New York, nestled between an Islamic center and a Kentucky Fried Chicken, a fit, elderly man known as Mr. P. runs an informal but tight-knit organization he calls the North Avenue Chess Club. When I first started hanging out there, the place looked like an abandoned pawnshop—clutter dominating 80 percent of the floor space, bric-a-brac worthy of an aspiring hoarder, plants that hadn't been watered since Milli Vanilli won a Grammy. At least the toilet flushed.

In chess, an inferior player will often find him- or herself in a miserable situation known as zugzwang, a turning point in the game where every possible move deteriorates the player's position. The player would prefer not to move—"pass" would be the best option were it allowed. It is not.

On the many occasions Mr. P. has put me in zugzwang—usually during an agonizing endgame when my pawns are blocked and my lonely king's been reduced to a senescent Lear on the heath—the feeling is familiar. Felicia and I spent the years after Sebastian's diagnosis in our own personal zugzwang, torn between the following set of bad options, all of which carried life-defining, and possibly life-ending, health risks for our baby boy.

1. **Live with it.** By maintaining the current regimen of
medications, environmental restrictions, and fetishistic
Clorox wiping and handwashing, we could minimize Sebastian's
odds of catching an infection through sheer force of discipline.
He'd likely get seriously sick once every couple of years anyway,
requiring weeks of hospitalization. We'd sometimes refer to this as
the Pinocchio option: our child could live, but not as a whole, free
boy—the disease would remain his invisible puppeteer. The
upside was obvious—he wouldn't have to endure the pain and risk
of a BMT. The downsides: an impoverished quality of life; the
cumulative toll exacted on the body by repeated infection; and
eventually, an emergent systemic resistance to the medications,
rendering them useless. Before this was all over, we'd meet several
adults with CGD and see how the Pinocchio option played out—
some appeared hale and hearty, others looked physically broken
and emotionally defeated. And of course, some patients never
make it to adulthood at all. We had no way to know how Sebastian
would end up.

2. **Transplant.** The upside: he could be cured of the disease and
live the rest of his life as a healthy child. Not just "not sick but
not well"—healthy. Environmentally unrestricted and
permanently emancipated from the bondage of his illness. The
downside: the possibility of a bad outcome during or after the
process. The minefield included the threat of organ failure from
the chemo; a failed engraftment of the donor cells; and/or the
ravages of graft-versus-host disease (GvHD), a condition specific
to transplantation in which the donor cells conclude the host's
body is a pathogen and attack it. Depending on the number and
severity of these problems, they could amount to nothing more
than a mild hiccup along the way to complete recovery; or they
could mean death in a pediatric intensive care unit. Permanent,

severe post-transplant health complications were also a
possibility—a transplant patient could wind up worse off than
he started.

3. **Wait for a breakthrough.** Sebastian's CGD was caused by a
   monogenetic mutation—that one misguided CYBB gene on the X
   chromosome. It was therefore an excellent candidate for gene
   therapy—there was but one lone troublemaker to repair. Gene
   therapy is getting a lot of press these days, but the original concept
   has been around since the seventies: modify a patient's DNA and
   reinsert it into his/her cells so that it will successfully transfer
   and then begin making the proper proteins to treat a disease.

For decades researchers around the globe have been hunting gene
therapy like a unicorn. The search for a safe and effective approach reliable enough to win FDA approval has consumed hundreds of millions of dollars. In recent years that massive effort has begun to bear
fruit. The year of Sebastian's diagnosis, 2012, saw a breakthrough with
the discovery that bacterial enzymes can be used to edit genes using
a remarkably effective, simple, and inexpensive technique called
CRISPR-Cas9. This technique has launched the so-called CRISPR
revolution—it's made gene editing so easy DIY CRISPR kits are now for
sale on Amazon for around $170, and today there are hundreds of on-
going gene therapy clinical trials. For CGD patients, they hold the
promise of curing the disease without many of the risks of a BMT. Less
chemotherapy would be required, and because the technique uses the
patient's own cells, graft-versus-host disease is a nonissue.

The NIH has been at the forefront of this research, and Dr. Malech
is among those leading the charge. Before the dawn of the CRISPR revolution, researchers had begun to develop and test other techniques
with cool names like TALENs and zinc finger nucleases. Malech

himself has been pursuing a technique using lentivirus vectors. Lentiviruses, of which HIV is the most famous example, are famously effective at delivering genetic information into the DNA of a host cell. Ingeniously, Malech and his colleagues are turning that deadly efficiency on its head, modifying the lentivirus to insert modified, disease-curing genes instead of HIV. Same great delivery system with a much more helpful payload.

It's easy for PWASK to find themselves mesmerized by the potential of these new techniques. The vision of a cure with all the upsides of a BMT and a much-diminished downside is a catalyst for magical thinking. *We'll just wait until gene therapy is approved*, the thinking goes, *it's right around the corner.*

"There's an argument for waiting [for gene therapy]," Malech had told us. "We know for sure that whatever treatments we'll be offering in five years, they'll be better than what we're doing now. But bear in mind—gene therapy has been 'just around the corner' for fifteen years."

Previous trials, he explained, cured the underlying condition as promised, but they were discontinued after patients developed leukemia a few years out. This possibility—that the genetically modified cells might cause cancer—can't be eliminated until "cured" patients are monitored for several years. As Malech explained, this presents one of the knottier questions of bioethics: How long do we need to observe you before you can feel safe?

"So much still needs to happen for the FDA to approve a CGD gene therapy," he said. "And even then, like many new treatments, it may only be approved for patients for whom nothing else has worked." Indeed, there's a consistent pattern in the writing of most news articles on gene therapy breakthroughs: lead with the anecdote of a miraculous cure from one of the trials, lay out the potential game-changing implications, then end with a series of deflating disclaimers about how far off an approved therapy really is. We indulged occasionally in the heady brew of gene therapy daydreaming, but when we came to our senses we recognized the folly of betting our child's life on so many things falling into place before his carriage turned into a pumpkin.

Malech had assured us we had time. We could take months, even years, to do our homework, explore the options, and arrive at a decision we could stand by. *When in doubt, gather data.*

One catch: there was danger in excessive dithering. The odds of a successful BMT diminish significantly after a patient turns five. If we waited for Sebastian to grow old enough to make an informed decision for himself (the "pass" option out of zugzwang at last!), we'd be narrowing his chances of making it.

We could neither weasel out of this decision nor delay it indefinitely. This call would be ours alone and we'd live with it forever. To make it, we'd need to find within ourselves what it takes to be a true adult: the strength to make decisions with profound and irreversible consequences under conditions of imperfect information. Outwardly, I was putting on a good front of stoic fortitude, but to myself I wondered— When the time came, would I be ready to act like a full-grown man?

As 2013 unfurled, Sebastian's health was holding steady. The drugs were working. He started walking at the precocious age of nine months and evinced a prodigious talent for pedaling his scooter around neighborhood sidewalks. People who met him couldn't believe he had a deadly illness. We wouldn't say anything until someone leaned in to touch him. At home, he'd taken such a shine to the strawberry costume he'd sported for his first Halloween he'd wear it all day, giggling as his big sister taught him to dance. His body was growing, his mind developing, his world expanding.

It was wonderful to put the endless hospitalizations of 2012 behind us. But as our baby grew bigger and stronger, it became that much harder to imagine putting such a thriving, happy child through a BMT.

That ambivalence is widespread, not only among CGD families but their doctors as well. "Many immunologists simply won't send CGD patients to transplant unless they have severe infections," said Malech. "It's the kind of disease where you say, "Prove to me you need it."

Disagreements about treatment can cause major domestic ruptures—recently, a CGD mother in Alaska had to fight her ex-husband in court to get her son admitted for transplant. The dad in that case simply didn't think it was worth the risk, and each side had medical evidence backing them up.

Felicia and I knew we had to make the decision unanimously, if only to make sure one of us couldn't blame the other if things went sour. For me it was easy to understand and accept the risks of transplant but harder to get my head around the logistics—uprooting ourselves to another city if necessary and committing at least a full year to the process. I was also troubled by mundane concerns such as the damage this could inflict on our finances and my career.

"I live in the real world, where I have to work," I mansplained to my wife, "and my work supports this family and our health insurance. We can't jeopardize that."

Felicia had no such qualms. "We need to do what is in Sebastian's best interest," she said. "Everything else will work out."

Within days of our return from NIH, she was scouring the Internet and working the phone, reaching out to patient groups like the Immune Deficiency Foundation, which in turn connected her with other CGD moms.

It was an immense comfort for her to commiserate and bond with other women who'd been navigating this excruciating situation for years, in some cases decades. Their emotional support was a life preserver. And yet, their advice only added to our confusion. One mother talked at length about how one of her two CGD sons was going strong well into his thirties without a BMT; she spoke more tersely about the other son, who'd died three years earlier. Some mothers described transplant as a miracle cure; others described it with regret as "the most horrible experience of my life." Some described managing the disease with meds as no greater a burden than managing other common conditions like diabetes; others described it as a doomed venture and blamed themselves for lacking the nerve to roll the dice on transplant. "The kids can seem normal for years . . . until suddenly they aren't."

Whether or not to transplant was only the first question; deciding *where* to transplant was a perplexing process all its own. We had to feel comfortable with both the process and the people. The list of choices wasn't overwhelming—transplants for leukemia are available at most major hospitals, but CGD transplants are a specialty performed at only about a dozen centers. The challenge was sifting through the data from each one and trying to evaluate the claims and reputations of respective transplanters—no easy task for a layperson.

The variety of transplant protocols has mushroomed in recent years. The "standard" model now competes with funky innovations like T-cell depletion and the Johns Hopkins haploidentical method, each with its own advantages and risks. Behind each technique stands a crusading transplanter, a personality type that, we learned, shares traits with the stereotypical start-up founder—inventive, committed, zealous. "The transplanters are nothing if not enthusiastic about their particular approach," Dr. Malech said with a half chuckle. "They're all quite convinced that what they are doing is the best."

Another factor complicating our decision—most hospitals are for-profit operations. Each transplant represents at least a million dollars' worth of business. The hospitals are thus incentivized to present impressive success rates, a stat they can juke by simply demurring to take on the hardest cases. What does your shooting percentage really mean if you're never attempting three-pointers?

Fumbling through this fog, we began scheduling phone calls and planning visits to the top transplant centers. The diagnostic odyssey of 2012 was to have a sequel: the treatment odyssey of 2013. Our quest had begun.

"Think of it like planning college visits for a high school senior," Felicia said one morning over a breakfast table littered with hospital brochures and medical studies.

"Mmmm," I grumbled, "more like the Magical Misery Tour."

Unfortunately, the two most convenient choices were off the table—New York's Memorial Sloan Kettering had little experience transplanting CGD patients, and the NIH in D.C. wasn't equipped to transplant children as young as Sebastian. Philadelphia was a promising option because the Children's Hospital of Philadelphia (CHOP) has an excellent reputation and my mom lived in Philly, so we could use her house as a home base. We arranged a visit with immunologist Kathleen Sullivan, a no-nonsense doctor who wasn't shy about giving straight answers. She would have done well in the military.

Without hesitation Sullivan told us to transplant as soon as possible. But CHOP's protocol involved a traditional, full-blast chemotherapy protocol using a harsh drug called busulfan. Before we went into that dark forest, we wanted to exhaust any less fearsome alternatives.

We flew across the country to meet with the transplanters at Seattle Children's. (The five-hour plane ride alone consumed two full boxes of Clorox wipes and ten ounces of Purell—a fuselage is a flying petri dish.) A mecca of bone marrow transplantation and home to many breakthroughs in the field, the center boasts a state-of-the-art pediatric unit with spacious, glass-walled patient rooms. The team there was conducting a tantalizing clinical trial with an alternate chemo drug called treosulfan, reputed to be gentler on the system but equally as effective as busulfan. We were taken with this prospect, and the thought of spending a year in Seattle, where several of my closest friends live, had an added appeal. We initiated the enrollment and screening process, but at the last minute, Dr. Malech waved us off the trial. He said something vague about waiting until Sebastian was closer to three or four, but later he said he'd harbored some doubts about Sebastian's chances of success in that protocol. In any event, as of this writing treosulfan has yet to receive FDA approval.

We continued to work through a list of august medical institutions, the pantheon of pediatric medicine: Cincinnati Children's Hospital, MD Anderson Cancer Center in Houston, Boston Children's Hospital. At the same time, we'd begun the parallel process of finding a match—a donor whose blood had a compatible typing with Sebastian's. Without a suitable match, the hunt for the ideal transplant center was an academic exercise.

The general public's exposure to bone marrow donation is built around made-for-TV moments when a cured patient gets a surprise visit from the lifesaving donor they've never met. The introduction is often emceed by a huggable celebrity like Emeril Lagasse.

That's the happy ending. The beginning and the middle don't make for great TV.

Blood typing for BMTs is not the same thing as typing for regular transfusions, the kind of typing the Red Cross does for local blood drives. That ABO classification system pertains to antibodies on the *red* blood cells and plasma. There are billions of type O people on the planet and even the rarest type—AB negative—is shared by millions. Potential donors aren't hard to find.

BMTs deal with the *white* blood cells of the immune system. These are matched by human leukocyte antigen (HLA) typing, which is much more complex. HLA type is determined by the combination of antigens and alleles found on ten separate loci on chromosome 6. The diversity among HLA types is staggering—there are trillions of possible combinations. A successful transplant depends on the donor and patient matching on at least eight out of the ten loci (nine and ten matched loci are always preferable, of course). Transplanting with an inadequately matched donor is a recipe for graft-versus-host disease. (Ignorance of this important point is why so many of the first transplant patients died; it is because of their deaths that we have learned what we know now.)

A donor search always begins with the patient's siblings. Due to their shared genes, a fully matched sibling will almost always guarantee a smoother transplant. Each child inherits half of the HLA type from each parent, so by simple Mendelian genetics the chances of a full sibling match are 25 percent. (Identical twins, of course, are guaranteed to match.) We got slapped by those odds in Philadelphia when Dr. Sullivan took a scraper to the inside of Lydia's cheek. She was not a match.

The news was crushing—another bad break. We'd envisioned our wonderful daughter, the source of so much light in our lives, angelically saving her little brother's life in a transcendent act of altruism, connecting them forever. Sullivan always roots for sibling matches, but she noted that at least we'd dodged another potential stressor: matched siblings often feel tremendous pressure for the transplant to succeed and an oppressive, lifelong guilt if it doesn't. Perhaps it was better to leave that burden off Lydia's slender shoulders.

With a sibling match ruled out, our attention pivoted to finding a matched unrelated donor—known in the biz as a MUD. For that we turned to the National Marrow Donor Program, and its Be the Match Registry, a database into which roughly fifteen million prospective donors have volunteered their sample cells. A moment here to reflect on the selflessness this involves: donating bone marrow is traditionally a much more involved process than simply donating blood (though

less intrusive techniques are evolving). An approved donor traditionally agrees to be admitted to a hospital and anesthetized, and then endure a procedure involving an incision and the insertion of a small
needle directly into the pelvic bone. For all this trouble, the donor has
no say over what happens next—you can't designate your marrow for
exclusive use by specific individuals or classes of patients. The propo-
sition is simple: all give, no take.

One of the curious and marvelous things about MUDs is that they
can come from any ethnic group or nationality. While shared ethnic
groups often share HLA types, it's possible for someone who looks
nothing like you, from a wholly separate gene pool, to be a perfect
match. This makes for those heartstring-plucking stories of strangers
from across the globe saving people they've never met and never would
meet—a Namibian could save a Canadian, an Afghan could save an
Argentine. Little reminders that compassion and generosity dot the
earth's surface like sprinkles on an ice cream scoop, that beneath our
divisive skins lie quirky bonds—of biology, of kindness—connecting
us at random.

The NIH typed Sebastian's blood and initiated the search. The
preliminary results were hopeful but not a home run. Five potential
MUDs popped up in the database, and while Felicia and I found that
promising we learned that some searches turn up hundreds or even
thousands of candidates. The difference-maker is the patient's ethnicity. Kids with parents of identical ethnic backgrounds typically
have more common HLA types, especially if the ethnicity is a population from which many people have registered as donors (it's still a new
and relatively unpopular thing in some parts of the world).

Kids of mixed ethnicity have it tougher. Their HLA type is usually
quite rare. Such was Sebastian's fortune. I'm 100 percent Latino, as my
Costa Rican mother is proud to remind me. Felicia is a mélange of
various European peoples, including the Finns. Given that those two

countries have small populations and have neither invaded nor immigrated to each other en masse, our son is likely one of very few living male *Homo sapiens* to have both Finnish and Costa Rican ancestors. In conversations about the great American melting pot, that's an uplifting story. In discussions about HLA matching it's a bummer. The kid's HLA type was as rare as his disease.

We talked this through with Dr. Malech when the results came back. "It's true you only have five potential matches," he reassured us, "but all it takes is one." We tried to stay positive, but as mentioned earlier, once you come up on the losing end of a 1 in 250,000 rare disease diagnosis, it's hard to believe the odds will ever play out in your favor.

Of the five potential donors, two lived in the United States, one was in Germany, one was in Latin America, and one in the Czech Republic. Felicia, who'd lived in Prague, zeroed in on the Czech. She quickly began imagining a Smetana-scored scene with our family and the donor running to each other's arms from opposite ends of the Charles Bridge and tearfully embracing at its midpoint. Then we'd all retire to a local pub for slivovitz, dumplings, and perhaps a surprise appearance by Emeril Lagasse, camera crew in tow.

Drilling down to determine if any of the potentials was a true match would take the NIH several more months. Each had to be contacted and then agree to come in for further testing. Not all do, especially those who register hoping to help a specific patient, only to learn later they weren't a match. As the process wore on with no news, my cousin Lee and some of Felicia's relatives kindly offered to organize donor drives in their spare time. They netted a few dozen registrants, but the chances of any one of them matching were infinitesimal.

Perhaps we'd get out of zugzwang through sheer happenstance—if no matched donor could be found, we might just have to live with the Pinocchio option regardless of what move we would have chosen. And that was starting to feel tolerable. Other CGD families were keeping their boys alive, some while living in remote locations hundreds of miles from any doctor with CGD expertise. For them the sporadic life-threatening infections were just the cost of doing business. If they could make a go of it, why not us?

At some point in the summer of 2013, as I was settling into that possibility, Felicia approached me with a radical idea, a plan C that blew my mind. "What if we had *another* child," she mused, "and took steps to make sure it would be a match for Sebastian?"

I swallowed a reflexive "Hell no!" and formulated a neutral response. "Took steps? How would that work?"

"We'd do IVF and then screen the embryos for one with the right HLA type." In theory this made sense—siblings had a 25 percent chance of matching; if we produced four viable embryos the odds would be in our favor for once.

I was struck dumb. It may be an iron law of our culture that today's parents are supposed to "do anything" to save the lives of their children, but the idea of creating life—a designer baby—for a purely instrumental purpose felt as perverted as slavery. From a bioethics perspective the notion wasn't as outrageous as Chinese-style organ harvesting—BMTs aren't the same as other organ transplants, since the donated body part grows back—but there was no denying that we'd be creating a human life expressly to extract his or her stem cells. And what would become of the nonmatching embryos? I'm not inclined to moral preening, but it gave me the willies.

And yet, other conscientious families have done it, even before it was possible to perform HLA typing in utero. Dawn, a mother from Georgia and a woman of deep faith, said she wrestled with the decision after she gave birth to a CGD boy in 1996. "I didn't want to be playing God," she told me, "but our pastor told me it was for good and not for bad. We decided to have a second baby and my faith was strong. I firmly believed I was going to have a healthy baby girl."

Sadly, that's not how it worked out for her family. Dawn got pregnant with another boy who'd inherited the disease. Two years later, she gave birth to a baby girl, born a CGD carrier and not a match.

Uncertain outcomes and ethical concerns notwithstanding, the thought of having a third child was terrifying in itself. The costs involved—exacted in time, money, and peace of mind—would have been a deal breaker for me even if all three kids were perfectly healthy. I knew myself and the situation well enough to know that there was no way we could juggle any more responsibility, much less assume the risk that this new baby might have unforeseen health issues of its own.

"You ever see those Olympic weight lifters who attempt a clean and jerk with more weight than their bodies can bear?" I asked Felicia from my side of the couch. "The ones who end up breaking their arm at the elbow live on NBC? I feel like I could turn into one of those guys any minute as it is." Once upon a time I'd dreamed of having a *big* family—five or six kids, a huge house out in the boonies. After a full year as a PWASK, I was ready to leapfrog the parenting years altogether and skip ahead to a quiet dotage.

Still, Felicia is a virtuoso in the art of persuasion. She could have gotten her way if she wanted it badly enough.

She didn't.

Our marriage may have been steady enough to take on an additional load of risk and responsibility in the early going. Sadly, we both knew, it had become as flimsy as a Jenga tower, and it was starting to teeter.

Chapter 7

A House Divided

Like many a man with cause to ponder the subject, I can't recall the precise moment my marriage began to unravel. Divorce can come in the wake of a dramatic singularity—say, the discovery of extensive backpage.com activity on an unsecured laptop—but in my experience relationships don't detonate as frequently as they decay.

By the summer of 2013, as we approached a full year as PWASK, it was clear the diagnosis itself had infected our marriage, spreading, damaging its vital organs. In our defense, we weren't unique. "Our patient families are a very vulnerable population," says John G. Boyle, the president of the Immune Deficiency Foundation. "This issue of not taking the time to tend to the marriage, of letting yourself get into a bad place, that essentially comes with the territory. And that goes for most relationships with other people who keep you centered—most of that goes out the window almost entirely."

Like many CGD parents, Felicia and I found that the disease sucked up so much time, money, and emotional bandwidth that it crowded out the opportunity to reinforce our relationship. "We were in survival mode," one mom told me. "We weren't a married couple anymore, we were just partners, working in shifts." "We just put so much focus on the kids that we lost any kind of connection with each other," said another.

Felicia and I were falling into the same trap. Even when there was no immediate crisis, talking about Sebastian's medical needs became a default conversation topic, a silence filler like the weather or real estate. Perhaps it didn't occur to us to interact the way we had in our enchanted pre-diagnosis days because they seemed like Shirley MacLaineish echoes of prior lives. In any case, we were directing our love at the kids more than at each other.

It's easy to say the stress made this disharmony inevitable, but recent research shows that most marriages are not, in fact, doomed to failure when they come under that strain of a child's chronic illness. Other CGD parents' accounts of the marital repercussions run the gamut—many couples, to their eternal credit, grew closer through their shared ordeal, refocusing their lives on family and appreciating each day together. Many others ran aground. The situation is never easy, but it is what you make of it.

I made it a mess.

To the casual observer, it looked like we were hanging tough. We formed a Facebook Group page to keep our inner circle looped in on our journey—if that was your sole source of information, you'd conclude we were marching forward with chests out and chins up. Picture-perfect PWASK.

It wasn't all an act, but even in our happiest moments we never achieved that state of rejuvenating euphoria we had with Lydia. Happiness in general had taken a back seat to our new sense of purpose—what we'd lost in fun we hoped to recoup in meaning.

The point of our existence, our solitary and overmastering goal, was always front and center, blinking in boldface the Terminator's mission objective on its retinal imaging display: MUST KEEP BOY ALIVE. This was a worthy and sacred goal.

Unlike the postapocalyptic setting of *The Terminator*, however, the rest of humanity hadn't been wiped out—on the contrary, everyone around us was proceeding merrily with abundant lives, some comically prosperous. Our friends had their troubles, but almost all their kids were healthy. While they were debating which fancy day care to apply for, we were wondering if Sebastian would ever be able to attend school at all. While they were vacationing in popular tourist destinations, we were traveling to transplant centers. Their aspirations for their kids were limitless; ours couldn't be more basic: survival. Our ceiling was their floor.

We knew so many people—PWASK and others—had it worse, and there were constant reminders to help us keep things in perspective. But behind our FB pics, a nasty feeling was calcifying in my mind as gradually and inexorably as a stalactite: we'd been cheated by life.

When my mind drifted into those dark places, I tried to tow it back with my favorite mantra—*Just focus on what's in front of you*—retargeting my attention on the mission objective: MUST KEEP BOY ALIVE. If only it were that simple.

Adhering to Dr. Malech's list of dos and don'ts had been challenging but straightforward during Sebastian's infancy; things grew ever more complex as he grew into a toddler. As his motor skills developed, he was grabbing everything he could and putting it into his mouth if it fit. Yikes. After he started walking he wanted ever more time outside the apartment, but much of the natural world, the green places we associate with beauty and harmony, was a hostile environment. Earth itself— the dirt, the grass—was a danger, one of the quiet tragedies that barricaded him inside his disease.

Other kids were just as hazardous. He'd see little boys at the playground and want to befriend them, but playdates, the cornerstone of socialization, were high-risk affairs that had to be planned with the meticulousness of the Reagan-Gorbachev Reykjavík Summit. If the other kid came down with a last-minute sniffle, the whole thing was scuttled.

Fortunately, Lydia loved her little brother deeply and enjoyed being his best and only friend. She helped him build a world of his own inside our four walls. When she was a two-year-old only child, a family friend had passed down a large box of wooden Thomas the Tank Engine toys—tracks, bridges, and of course the locomotive characters. Lydia had taken to laying them out on the floor of the living room and acting out little scenes in the voices of the different characters. By the time Sebastian was born she'd moved on to other entertainments, so she bequeathed the train set to her brother.

Sebastian took it to another level. After his sister showed him around the Island of Sodor's narrative universe, he quickly developed a passion for Thomas that was as much an effective coping technique as it was a childhood obsession. For a little boy who wasn't allowed much contact with his peers, the engines Thomas, Percy, Gordon, James, and Emily became his most intimate and trusted companions for years. It was both touching and heartbreaking to watch the innocent child optimize his constrained circumstances.

Felicia spent hours each day on the floor playing with him. She'd taken our mission directive to heart, and for her that meant sacrifice. Her career as a PR consultant had gone supernova after she'd guided a dot-com start-up from infancy to IPO, but after Sebastian's diagnosis she had to dial her business down to devote herself to his care. It was both noble and necessary, but the amputation of that second income hobbled our household finances, adding another layer of stress. "I'm worried that you're going to be furious about my personal expenses now that I'm not making money," she warned me, "and I'm terrified of being totally dependent on you."

Still, we could have managed all of it—the money issues, the medical worries, the environmental restrictions, the social costs, the shrinking of our prefrontal cortexes, all the thorny hardships of parenting on the edge—had we had more effective methods of dealing with our pain.

Buoyed by her faith, Felicia did a valiant job keeping her spirits up in front of the kids, mindful that the family would mirror her energy and emotional state. Yet there were times—when I was at work, Lydia was at school, and Sebastian was with a babysitter—when she would lock herself in our bedroom and sob till her throat hurt.

I lacked such powers of self-control. By now my stoic façade had shattered irreparably. My emotional palette was dominated by three primary colors: sadness, fear, and anger.

Sadness was constant, but it was also the easiest of the three to handle. It manifested in spontaneous crying jags and an overall sense of heaviness, a feeling that I was wearing a full suit of thick clothing, like a fireman's turnout gear. This is apparently one of the telltale signs of depression, correlating with decreased serotonin and dopamine levels in the brain.

The heavy feeling wasn't only in my head. Like many people suffering from depression, I was overeating—I come from a long line of fat people and if I'm not careful I can struggle to squeeze into thirty-six-inch-waist jeans. That's where I was now—opting for sweatpants at home, wearing ties less frequently at work to avoid asphyxiation by buttoned shirt collar.

The fear had a different profile. Sometimes it was only quiet background noise; sometimes it was deafening. At the lower quantum levels, it was easy to recognize, tolerate, and ignore. When it peaked, it was dark and dominating to the point of inducing paralysis. I felt it physically as a scaly, electrified claw reaching up from the top of my stomach and grabbing hold of my spine with its talons. I nicknamed this intense anxiety "the Dragon," the embodiment of the chaos that had spread from the outside world into my nervous system. Its power was overwhelming, rekindling my insomnia for days and driving me close to what pretherapeutic cultures defined as demonic possession.

Anger was the cheap antidote for both the fear and the sadness. The adrenaline rush, the ego inflation, the feeling of (momentary) empowerment that comes when one morphs from Bruce Banner into the Hulk—it can be an almost orgasmic high, and it can grow into an addiction.

Work had become something of a refuge. There was a semblance of order to counterbalance the churning entropy that defined the rest of my life. I tried to keep a Berlin Wall between the two worlds, but reality kept seeping through the cracks, and as it did my composure slipped.

A chronic irritability set in; incidents and semi-successful apologies started piling up. In some cases it was an eruption of hot temper—a raised, profane voice, often directed at subordinates for some perceived incompetence, at peers for some perceived territorial encroachment, or at superiors for some perceived bureaucratic myopia. In many others it was what I might call "cold temper"—a tropism to arrogance, the overmastering need to be clever, a tendency to weaponize my erudition. The shrinks call this "grandiosity." The rest of the world calls it being an asshole.

At home the waters grew choppier by the month, churning eventually into a permanent hurricane season. Felicia and I shared clarity of purpose but we lacked clarity of approach. Malech's list of no-no's didn't address countless marginal situations where we had to rely on our own judgment. Mulch was a major threat, but could Sebastian run through a playground surfaced with wood chips? Sandboxes were out of the question, but could he play at the beach?

Was a rash on his face worth a visit to the pediatrician? A sniffle lasting more than two days? A scrape on the knee from the head of a floorboard nail?

Our concerns ratcheted up a notch when it became clear Sebastian wasn't acquiring speech skills at a normal pace. Lydia had shot up the learning curve at his age, her operative vocabulary expanding as fast as ten words a day; at fourteen months Sebastian was still stuck on a handful of duo-syllabic utterances. We heard "mama" and "dada" frequently and "passy" for pacifier. Beyond that, not much.

Was there now an emergent cognitive issue layered on top of the immune deficiency? Did we require the diagnostic services of a neurologist? Was speech therapy in order, and, if so, when should it commence?

Each of these decisions big and small was open for discussion and thus an opportunity for disagreement. With the stakes so high, it was easy for those disagreements to become arguments. And as the grind of our situation wore on, shriveling the dendrons in our respective prefrontal cortexes, those arguments grew increasingly frequent. And caustic.

"That's a common flavor of marital disruption," said Boyle. "One parent will do the equivalent of a lockdown, the other will say it's being taken too far and start making accusations of Munchausen by proxy."

While the tension was escalating, Felicia was dealing with a chronic fatigue we'd later learn was common among CGD carriers. Occasionally it caused her to forget things or mix up something that needed to be done for Sebastian or Lydia. This would provoke me, the one with the temper issue, to make some snarky comment or put-down. She'd respond with a remark about how I wasn't doing enough or appreciating her sacrifices. With us both on edge, the air was always combustible and such skirmishes could quickly devolve into the Battle of Grozny. I'd imply she was stupid; she'd imply I was evil. Sometimes we did more than imply.

Inevitably I'd beg forgiveness and promise to do better. But as the African proverb goes: the axe forgets, the tree remembers. With each lacerating encounter, we grew further apart.

"I feel like I'm on my own here," she said over tapas at one of our stillborn date night dinners, "both from an emotional and practical standpoint. I feel like I'm taking care of *three* children."

"If I'm such a burden, perhaps I can arrange for you to *really* experience being alone for a while. Then you'll have a baseline to measure against."

"If you want to go, go. I guess you were lying when you said, 'For better, for worse, in sickness and in health.'"

"Mmmmm. I just figured it would be at least a fifty-fifty split between better and worse. *This* was not part of the bargain."

Such corrosive spats slowly became the norm; some are too shameful to include here, many others just too tedious and repetitive. Deep down, Felicia resented that I still had a career and was sustaining a life outside the disease. Deep down, I resented that the situation originated in her family's gene pool. Deep down can be an ugly place. "Once the blame game ramps up, it gets complicated fast," said Boyle.

The glue holding the family together was Lydia. At five years old, engaged and cheery, her love was a fire hose. She was now fully aware of her brother's situation—to the point that she'd strain to swallow coughs and sneezes, a telltale *khck* sound coming from her throat every time—but instead of resenting the extra attention he got, she was eager to participate in his care. Without prompting she'd help tuck him into bed, remind us it was medicine time, and assist with diaper changes and baths. Mostly she was a great friend—not only to Sebastian but also to her parents.

An August vacation was supposed to turn things around and give us a fresh start. We rented a small house on one of Maine's countless fractal peninsulas. Mercedes, our nanny, couldn't be away from her own kids, so we arranged for one of Sebastian's babysitters, a quiet Filipina woman named Maria, to join us so Felicia could have a break.

The rental house had a fireplace and, as it still gets nippy up there in the summer, I threw some logs on one night and we gathered around the hearth. This was one of Sebastian's first fireplace experiences, and, curious child that he was, he toddled right up to the flames when I approached to add some kindling. The first time it happened I calmly asked Maria to keep him at a safe distance (the dead wood alone was an infection hazard). She marched him off to another room, but five minutes later he was back, putting his hand on the fireplace's glass door. I repeated, in a lower voice and without any trace of a smile, that she must keep him away from the flames.

The third time it happened, I exploded. *"GET . . . THE KID . . . THE FUCK . . . AWAY . . . FROM THE FIRE!"*

Maria retreated into her bedroom in tears and closed the door. Felicia went in to comfort her and came out with murder in her eyes. I tried to apologize, but that bridge was torched. Maria sat in stony silence the whole ride back to New York. We dropped her off at the E train, and at the top stair of the station entrance she turned and said sweetly in Tagalog-accented English, "Thank you for trip. I very happy."

She blocked our number that night. We never heard from her again.

Felicia was still simmering as we got home and unpacked. She was itching for a fight, and when she discovered I'd brought some cannabis cookies on the trip, she strode into the kitchen as I was grabbing a snack and stood there, glowering in silence.

"What *now*? What? . . . I swear to God, when you stare at me like that without talking, I can hear your tail rattle."

Then she launched a one-woman Tet Offensive, accusing me of endangering the children. *"POT COOKIES? Seriously? Sebastian could have eaten one of those things! What kind of father are you?"*

That cut deep. Call me ugly or insult my mom, but an indictment of my commitment to Sebastian, after all we'd been through, was the ultimate provocation. Unhinged, my resultant rage matched Rumpelstiltskin's when he didn't get the baby. It was scary. When the smoke cleared, Felicia commenced an extended period of silent treatment. I was banished to the couch and shunned like a leper. For a week my phone calls went straight to voicemail. When my wife finally spoke to me, it was to introduce the D-word into the vocabulary of our relationship.

Many a CGD mom has gotten divorced post-diagnosis and, to hear them tell it, the split is tough but tolerable. Felicia had heard enough of those testimonies to believe she could swing it if she had to. She demanded a brief separation and, as it happened, one had been scheduled already. Every summer she took the kids up to her mom's place in Ontario for a few weeks. Soon she was packing their stuff. Sebastian's tiny socks, Lydia's favorite stuffed animals, the medicines, Thomas and some of his closest friends—I watched as they all went into a big black Samsonite I'd once purchased as a prop for a story about a girl who'd been abducted out of a Miami hotel stuffed in a suitcase of the same make. Watching my wife cram toiletries into the side pockets and zip the suitcase closed, I glimpsed a little preview of how the last goodbye would play if we called it quits. The foretaste of failure on a colossal scale. All I'd ever wanted, lost.

"I need some space and I need some time," she said. "But mostly I need to know that you're going to do what it takes to get yourself back to the husband I need you to be."

I saw them off in a taxi. Two enthusiastic, long tight hugs from the kids; a begrudged third from my wife, short and loose, to keep up appearances. Then I went back up to the apartment. Devoid of wife and children, the place was a Joni Mitchell lyric—bed too big, frying pan too wide. I'd assumed the respite from the burdens of family life would be a cherished furlough, but within minutes of an On Demand *Breaking Bad* episode I began to miss them beyond the power of all distraction. Not just the family, the burdens too.

The heavy sad feeling returned, a bowling ball in my belly.

She was right. This couldn't continue. Something had to change.

"I'm inclined to suggest a surround-the-football approach."

This was my friend Dan Harris, noted newsman, author, and meditator, dispensing cautiously worded advice over pasta downtown. It was about a week after Felicia had left with the kids; and after I'd given him an unsparing overview of my domestic situation, he was beginning to understand why I looked so miserable and defeated.

I'd expected him to launch into a hard sell on mindfulness meditation, a practice for which he's become a well-known champion. To my surprise, he was advising me to embrace *any* modality of treatment or self-help that might make a difference, all at once if need be. Anything from art therapy to yoga—as many as I could stand at one time.

"You really think that will do much good?" I pressed. Together we'd worked on a series of stories debunking *The Secret* and James Arthur Ray and other self-help gurus. This come one, come all attitude seemed out of step with his thinking.

"I have no idea if it will really help you wrestle with your demons," he answered. "But as I understand it, your main objective is to improve your marriage. And in my experience, women give points for effort."

So I went with Dan to the Insight Meditation Center on the West Side. "I was concerned I was sending you into an environment you'd find incredibly annoying," he'd say later. "The place looks like the living rooms of the progressive parents of my childhood friends—ferns, Zen art, Buddha statues. I thought you'd walk out had I not been there."

Instead, I left my introductory session feeling soothed, serene, and unjudged, in touch for the first time in a long time with what the instructor called our "natural nobility."

Over the course of the next several months, I committed myself to the practice—meditating every morning and going back to IMC once a week for an instructional seminar that included extended group "sits" and talks from an appointed speaker/teacher. The center, as it turned out, was across an air shaft from a popular Zumba studio; our sacred silence floated over the calorie-burning hits of Daddy Yankee, Pitbull, and Lil Jon.

Of the many helpful lessons of the teaching, none was as compelling and easy to practice as the concept of *metta*, the Sanskrit word translated as "loving-kindness." Essentially it means meditating on the wish that all creatures experience happiness, wellness, and peace, not just those who fall within our tribal social circles and not excluding ourselves. I worked this into my meditations, and then, at the recommendation of an experienced practitioner, I started mentally wishing loving-kindness on every living thing my gaze settled upon as I walked the streets of New York. The young cuff-linked hedge funder loudly talking into his phone about the killing he'd made shorting the Twitter IPO; the audibly flatulent dog that helped his panhandling owner earn $200 a day just for sitting in Grand Central, if the *New York Post* was to be believed; the Lululemoned divorcee leaving the Columbus Avenue Equinox—fifty bucks says her plastic surgeon also does Lenin's corpse—I envisaged a warm loving-kindness radiating outward from my body and engulfing them all.

The calming power of meditation made me marginally easier to be around—most notably, it helped curb my temper—but it was no panacea. That realization arrived later that fall, when two small white dots appeared near Lydia's left underarm. They didn't go away. Then they grew; first merging, then growing to a silver dollar–sized ellipse of depigmented flesh. After a visit to Edelstein the pediatrician and then to a dermatologist, it was confirmed—vitiligo.

Thanks to meditation, the Dragon had been hibernating for a few months. With the delivery of this news he awoke and grasped my spine with his electrified iron claw. Reassurances that this could turn out to be a minor case that wouldn't spread much further, that a prescription ointment was likely to help, meant nothing. All I could see, whether my eyes were open or closed, was my innocent daughter's beautiful face disfigured by yet another rare, untreatable condition. The anxiety roared through my head like the engine of an Airbus A380. I didn't sleep for days—the catastrophizing was making the worst-case scenario real in my head, and the emotional response was crippling.

I turned with in-case-of-emergency-break-glass haste to my mindfulness training. Surely its moment had arrived. As I sat in my living room, trying to subdue the Dragon, I succeeded instead in tuning out all my other thoughts *except* the one that was dominating my mind: *DISFIGURED DAUGHTER*. Essentially, I'd cleared out space in my mental cargo hold and made more room for the surging waves of anxiety to flood in.

Someone else has said that for someone in a state of crisis, meditation can be an act of cruelty. That may be putting it strongly, but at that moment the Eightfold Path wasn't doing much to liberate me from suffering. The Buddha, as legend has it, abandoned his wife and baby son to achieve nirvana—I take that as an indicator that dedication to enlightenment doesn't mix easily with the pressures of parenthood.

I didn't give up on meditation. I still try to sit every day for at least a few minutes, twenty if I'm being good. I believe Dan is correct: you can count on it making you "10 percent happier." And, as he says, "It works better as a prophylaxis than as a Band-Aid." If, however, you're in such intense pain you really need to get 50 or 100 percent happier in a hurry, additional methods may be required.

So I went to the gym. Throwing myself into a hard-core diet, sobriety kick, and exercise regimen, I dropped twenty-five pounds in three months. Aside from earning compliments on my "new body," maintaining a clean lifestyle restored a sense of order and control. The strict asceticism was a good complement to the meditation—I was proving to myself that I was not a slave either to my appetites or my emotions.

All that clean living was wonderful but it wasn't much fun. Yummy food is one of life's great pleasures; so is a mellow buzz. All of which is to say, at a certain point I got sick of being so healthy. The predawn treadmill runs became less frequent, the pepperoni pizza binges became less rare. I'd snap back when things got out of control, but a clear pattern emerged—the pendulum swinging between self-discipline and self-indulgence, the weight from 185 to 225. If Oprah could accept that, so could I.

Then there was the therapy. For a year, at Felicia's behest, I saw a shrink, who quickly diagnosed me as a recalcitrant and mediocre patient. I wasn't coming in good faith, she suspected, going through the motions but unwilling to open up. In turn, I thought the process was something of a fraud. Her response to every problem I raised was a reflexive "Mmmm . . . and how did *that* make you feel?" That approach might work for many, but aside from earning me some of Dan's aforementioned brownie points with Felicia, I can't say it did much good.

Couples therapy was another matter. Felicia, who's always been more hospitable to self-help in all its forms than I, was amenable to a series of regular sessions with a Catholic therapist named William Lent we'd met during our pre-Cana, the intro-to-marriage seminar the Church requires of all couples planning to marry in the faith.

A slender, bespectacled man who looked like a cross between Stephen King and Willem Dafoe, Lent assured us we'd both have a chance to speak and be heard, but that he would direct the discussion—setting boundaries to prevent things from going China syndrome like our arguments at home.

A sampling of Lent's notes from the sessions, which included direct quotes, paint an accurate picture of how things went.

Miguel: I feel like I'm always on trial with you.

Felicia: You can't understand my insecurity or my fear.

Miguel: I don't want this to be another bitch session.

Felicia: Our situation is hopeless.

William: How can you find ways to love each other in the midst of what you're going through?

Felicia: I don't want to be reasoned with. I want to be joined in my feelings.

Miguel: I'm doing close to the best I can do, and I need that acknowledged. She keeps moving the goalposts.

William Note to self: M is in so much pain, and I can't help him get to it. Need to help him have compassion for himself; invite F to do likewise.

Some bleak stuff there, but eventually we started loving more than litigating. The help was indeed helping. The arguments became less frequent and intense. The needle was moving out of the red zone, where the relationship is fully militarized and every questionable remark or deed is interpreted in the most negative light, and into the green zone, where we once again saw each other as a team and began to grant each other the benefit of the doubt. (I think I got those terms from some couples book I can't presently name.)

This was more than talk. All that work—on ourselves, on our relationship—underwent a major stress test at the end of the year. Right as Christmas was rolling around, Sebastian came down with another infection. United against a common bacterial enemy, Felicia and I shelved our squabbles and focused on what was *really* important. (This became a pattern and eventually a shared dark joke—if Sebastian was sick, Felicia and I declared a truce. If we were fighting, that was a good sign in its own twisted way—it meant Sebastian was healthy enough for us to "afford" that "luxury.")

With the composure of a veteran firefighter responding to an alarm, Felicia packed the extra changes of clothes, medicines, and food for what could be an extended hospital stay. "Never go to an ER hungry," she advised. "It just makes everything worse."

For the first time in months, the updates on our Facebook Group page carried bad medical news. The entries from that time are illuminative.

December 6—Miguel

On Friday Sebastian had a successful surgery and was discharged hours later. . . . This abscess was smaller than his previous ones, so the incision was similarly small and hopefully the recovery time will be similarly quick.

The other noteworthy thing about this time around is that our general levels of anxiety, stress, and anguish have been noticeably diminished compared to the last time. Why? Well, we now know what we're dealing with, we're familiar with the hospital and its procedures, and most important, through the practices of mindfulness and prayer we've learned how to avoid that gravitational pull toward doomsday thinking that sets the brain on a continuous feedback loop of fear and pain. We are not stoics—we don't simply ignore suffering and tell the world thank you, sir, may I have another? We believe suffering must be acknowledged and felt, but we cannot let it dominate or cripple us. . . .

December 6—Felicia

Dear Friends and Family,

Thank you for your kind words, thoughts, and prayers. As Miguel wrote, we both were somehow buoyed during this hospital visit. In addition to our efforts to be mindful and prayerful in situations like these, we felt your love and support, which helps so much. As for Sebastian, it was certainly painful and scary for him at times, but he handled it like a trooper.

We are grateful to you for keeping little Sebastian in your prayers. It is going to be a long journey, but we take comfort in knowing that you're with us.

Love, F.

This Hospitalworld visit was so much less traumatizing than our prior trips, we felt our relationship had evolved to the point where we no longer needed the therapy and we discontinued the sessions. Lent said that was a bad idea. Time would prove him right.

By the spring of 2014 the Manhattan apartment had become claustrophobically cramped. Both kids had accumulated so much stuff their shared bedroom was basically one large closet with two sleeping surfaces. Sebastian still spent much of his time sequestered indoors and it felt cruel to keep him in such a small enclosure. And despite the countless joys we'd shared there, the apartment was now also crammed with unpleasant memories. In Felicia's words, "It began to feel like a trap." We were ready for a change.

We wound up in a lovely suburb in Westchester, but getting there was a disaster. The psychological trauma of moving is well established and between the stresses of putting our place on the market, wrestling with co-op boards and lawyers, and packing and purging, my mental fortitude and our marriage started backsliding.

By now Felicia had concluded that whatever improvements I'd made with the other modes of self-help, they needed a boost. She insisted I go on medication. I'd resisted the suggestion for years, as the notion of surrender to psychopharmacology cut against my machismo-shaped image of my own brain. But this time her demand was nonnegotiable.

That's how I arrived at the Park Avenue office of Dr. Rachel Moore, an unflappable psychiatrist whose name I've replaced because she didn't want to go on the record. Dr. Moore has some withering reviews online—"condescending and insulting," "waste of my money," "impatient, dismissive"—but I took her icy, patrician mien as well-intentioned tough love. In any case, I wasn't in the market for empathy or understanding. I just needed a fix. After an hour of candid conversation, I departed with scripts for the low-dose antidepressant Wellbutrin and a powerful schedule-IV antianxiety drug called Klonopin.

I'd heard of "Captain K" before, as several of my friends and co-workers swore by it. In fact, during the height of Sebastian's 2012 hospitalizations, a colleague had slipped me half a tab with an assuring smile. "Try it," she said like Carroll's Caterpillar. "It helps you deal." They should put those words on the bottle.

Dr. Moore considered my insomnia the most urgent issue, so her initial prescribed dose was strong enough to turn me into an extra from *The Walking Dead*. My nerves quieted and I got the sleep, but my consciousness downshifted to a steady stupor. Colleagues began asking what had taken the light out of my eyes.

I headed back to Dr. Moore and complained that at the current dosage my brain felt manifestly slower. "Have you considered," she replied, "that perhaps it's a *good* thing for your brain not to run so fast?" Still, she dialed the dosage back by half, eventually to an as-needed basis. As the Wellbutrin started paying dividends the following month, those needs became less frequent and pressing.

All the elements of the surround-the-football approach—the workouts, the sobriety, the therapy, the meditation, the meds—became part of what I loosely called my Program. I've never felt I was cheating by hopscotching around to different modalities of treatment, combining them improvisationally or sampling them cafeteria style. In fact, I've come to believe that the mind requires a variety of different tools to fight off psychological assault, much like the body's immune system requires its diverse army of cells to fight off different forms of infection. To this day I've found that unless I'm doing *some* combination of practices to maintain this mental immune system, the state of my marriage will deteriorate. While this polytherapous attitude may be the essence of half-assing it, while others may have achieved dramatically better results through other means, at least I learned how to restore enough order in my head to stay functional, and I haven't lost the greatest, truest coping aid I've ever come across—the love of my wife. If I've gained any expertise, it is in the field of *adequacy*.

Chapter 8

Cheever Country

....

We choreographed our tactical retreat to the burbs to coincide with Lydia's kindergarten graduation. After exploring dozens of towns in New Jersey and Long Island, we settled on Larchmont in Westchester County, a beautiful, affluent, and monochromatic community with great schools, a charming beach, and hideously inflated real estate prices. We could only afford a small house, but the "cozy" three-bedroom we landed in checked a lot of boxes—a finished basement for the kids and their container ship of toys, proximity to the train, a yard with a swing set. I bought a used Subaru Outback, the first vehicle I'd owned in twenty years. Welcome to Cheever country.

In Larchmont the sanitation truck comes three times a week, and the novelty of this marvelous municipal service never wore off. Lydia would often catch me on pickup mornings looking out the window at the burly men feeding garbage to their green metal mastodon, savoring the sight in silent awe. To her I looked like an Amazonian tribesman struck dumb by the magic of modernity, but my feeling was one of longing, not wonder. Bag trash, curb bag, watch truck haul it off—if only all life's problems could be thrown out with such simplicity . . . and finality.

Other alleviations abounded: housing, transportation, cleanliness, noise. Freed from the hassles of city life, on the good days my whole body felt like my upper arm does after the blood pressure cuff deflates. The conformity of the social scene was a drag, but we knew that going in. We hesitated to let our new neighbors in on our big family secret, but after we made a respectable first impression we eventually disclosed and embraced our identity as "that family." We assembled a team for an Immune Deficiency Foundation walk; we launched online Be the Match donor drives; we persisted with the uplifting updates on Facebook.

On the surface Sebastian's health was holding steady, so it was easy to maintain a brave face. In January 2015 we notched a full year with no hospitalizations. To the naked eye he was a loving, happy kid. He still didn't say much—his pet catchphrase was "I don't want to talk"—but Felicia got him qualified for publicly funded speech therapy and it seemed to do some good. His obsession with *Thomas & Friends* grew in proportion to his expanding collection of trains and tracks, which is where much of my disposable income went to be disposed. And as with any child, his personality evolved in funky, unexpected directions. Unlike his extrovert sister, Sebastian could be reclusive and overcautious, but in certain regards he expressed his will and his taste boldly. Notably, he developed a keen sense of fashion: he refused to leave the house without a hip newsboy cap; he wouldn't go to bed unless attired in freshly laundered matching pajamas; he insisted that his socks be slid onto his tiny feet with no bunching or misalignment. The word "perfect" went into heavy rotation in his limited operative vocabulary.

Extended stints of calm lulled us into the magical thinking he could live like this forever—but the medications and protections could do only so much. Our son had the most severe form of CGD—zero neutrophil function. He was getting by with a papier-mâché constitution. We kept him out of the hospital, but his growth was decelerating. Every checkup, he slid a few percentiles down the chart, and every few months there'd be some strange issue that had us on the hotline to Dr. Malech at the NIH. A weird rash appeared on his face. He'd get strange warts that wouldn't go away. His complexion went pallid and he needed treatment for anemia. And one Christmas, on account of a small internal cyst behind his right knee, he started hobbling around like Tiny Tim. Each issue eventually resolved, but only after frantic calls, a series of tests, and weeks on some additional medicine or ointment.

These oddities were layered on top of the usual colds and sniffles any child gets as the acquired immune system acclimates to the world and builds up antibodies to the countless viruses that cross our paths every day. CGD patients can fight off viruses like any normal kid—the neutrophil has nothing to do with those—but we had to be on guard for the telltale symptoms of a serious *nonviral* infection against which Sebastian was defenseless—a high fever and a persistent cough *without* an accompanying runny nose. (Dr. Malech explained that snot is a sign of viral infection—in other words, a good sign.) We dodged that bullet for years, but as Sebastian's health cycled up and down, we grew concerned that the peak of the most recent up was imperceptibly lower than the one before. Like a solvent company whose stock is on a gradual but irreversible decline—say GE from 2016 to 2018—the long-term trend line was unmistakable.

The chart of our marriage exhibited a similar periodicity and slope. Months of domestic tranquility—sustained by my Program and punctuated by genuinely wonderful, loving moments—would mask an accreting residue of inner pain—hers or mine or both. Then an argument would erupt, typically over something trivial—the absentminded purchase of nonorganic eggs (my sin) or the misplacement of a bill or check (hers)—and it would escalate until one of us (usually me) lost control and said something beyond the pale. A threat of divorce came next, followed by a period of silent and icy cohabitation with minimal interaction—we dubbed it roommate mode. Thankfully cold war is exhausting (just ask the Soviets) and eventually we'd slide into a budding glasnost and then, finally, a reconciliation with the promise to talk through our differences more reasonably next time.

Rinse and repeat, with each iteration of the cycle incrementally eroding the foundation of our relationship. On one memorable occasion, Felicia absconded with the kids and spent the night at a hotel. Many other incidents—the ones I don't want our kids reading about— have been left out of this text. Bottom line: all the programs, pills, and prayers couldn't reverse the destructive toll the disease was taking on our family.

There was one exit door—cure via BMT—but it was slipping out of reach. None of the five potential matched donors identified in the original database search turned out to be viable matches. A second, updated search, presumably including all the friends and relatives we'd registered, yielded nothing. "I don't know why we keep hitting roadblocks," Felicia said. "Why is God making this so hard for us?"

A field of intrepid transplanters was eager to work its medical magic on our son, but without a viable donor, the daring mission could not be launched, much less accomplished. We had some of the most advanced minds in medical science on our side, people who'd devoted their lives to helping families like ours. There was nothing they could do.

With one exception.

In a state-of-the-art lab at Duke University Hospital in Durham, North Carolina, a woman I'd never met was about to change our lives. Standing barely five feet, her head framed by tight short curls and librarian glasses, she inspired comparisons to Yoda, and in her field she enjoys equivalent stature.

Her name is Dr. Joanne Kurtzberg, and her career has been dedicated to breakthrough innovations in transplantation using stem cells harvested not from bone marrow but from a source once discarded as medical waste: umbilical cord blood (UCB).

Growing up in New York, Kurtzberg worked with severely autistic children before entering medical school and specializing in pediatrics and hematology/oncology. Like doctors Herzog and Malech, she was drawn intellectually and emotionally to the hardest cases. "I've always been attracted to difficult-to-solve problems," she said, "the kids who weren't curable, who required extraordinary measures."

It was not until the eighties, decades after the first BMT trials, that umbilical cord blood made its debut in the field of stem cell transplantation. Kurtzberg was part of the team that performed the key studies in lab mice, and then the first human transplant in 1988. Kurtzberg herself brought in the patient. Like Sebastian, he was a little boy with a rare and deadly disease; Dr. Kurtzberg reports that, as of this writing, he's a healthy married man in his thirties.

As the successes with umbilical cord blood multiplied, Kurtzberg founded the Carolinas Cord Blood Bank and built the Duke Pediatric Blood and Marrow Transplantation Program, saving thousands of lives while publishing hundreds of research papers.

What makes cord blood special? For starters, UCB cells are easy to collect: they're extracted from the umbilical cord at birth without disturbing the mother or the baby, a method much less intrusive than the arduous process of getting bone marrow cells from the pelvis of a human donor. And they be can be cryogenically preserved for decades.

They are also pure—unlike cells from a matched related or unrelated donor, UCB cells have never been exposed to illness or other environmental factors. They are pristine.

They are also "amiable"—UCB donor cells have been proven to get along better with their hosts; graft-versus-host disease occurs less frequently. The reason is another mystery of immunology. "Think about pregnancy," Kurtzberg told me. "The fetus is made up of genetic material from mother and father, so the fetus and the mother *should* identify each other as foreign presences and react accordingly [as mutual antagonists]. Yet that doesn't happen. The baby doesn't reject mom and mom doesn't reject the baby.

"It's an immunologic phenomenon, and it's carried over to cord blood cells. There's a lot of things going on in there, not all of them understood. We think T-cells in the cord blood can recognize a foreign thing, but then they forget. It's not a defect, it's a question of maturation. They just don't react to foreign things as they would normally if they were fully matured [as they are in bone marrow]. We think that's the reason we see less GvHD [with cord blood transplants]."

The promise of a smooth post-transplant experience was a strong selling point, but the real reason cord blood transplants are lifesavers for families like ours is that the cells are profoundly *malleable*. The donor unit doesn't have to be as closely matched as it does when transplanting with bone marrow cells from a matched unrelated donor. For mixed race/ethnicity kids like Sebastian, with exceedingly rare HLA blood typing, this makes all the difference. Recall that when using bone marrow stem cells, the transplanters are looking to match ten genetic loci for adequate HLA compatibility. With cord blood stem cells, it's only six. We'd spent years scouring the globe for a MUD, with nothing to show for it. Kurtzberg found a handful of viable UCB donor units within days.

Why doesn't everyone go this route? Traditionally, UCB transplants aren't an option for adults because the cell count in a UCB unit is too low to achieve engraftment in a patient of that size. (A minimum cell-count-per-kilogram ratio is required for success.) Today, double-unit transplants are now being done on some adult patients, but the procedure is still primarily for small kids. Also, cord blood transplants usually require the most severe regimen of chemotherapy conditioning, which many people rationally choose to avoid. And then there's the one-shot problem—when transplanting cells from a human donor you can always go back and get more if you need to; with UCB you blow through the entire unit. There's no going back for more. You either succeed or you return to square one with another donor unit, and the chances of a second transplant succeeding after a failed first attempt plummet by 50 percent.

Our choices had been reduced to this: take our chances with a cord blood transplant or take our chances living with the condition. We'd tried the latter and after walking that tightrope for three years the prospects of doing so indefinitely were grim. After a consultation with Dr. Malech, he arranged an introduction to Dr. Kurtzberg and in April 2015, Felicia and Sebastian boarded a southbound Amtrak and headed to Durham for yet another meet and greet with yet another visionary transplanter—the Jedi matron.

Felicia fell in love with North Carolina the moment she rolled Sebastian's stroller off the platform in downtown Durham. It wasn't just the lush, life-affirming scenery, the relaxed attitude, or the Southern hospitality. It was the sense of *belonging*. Duke has such a large footprint in Durham and the hospital draws so many patients from around the world that medical tourism is a significant chunk of the local economy. It's a PWASK mecca. At any given time, there are as many as fifty families with kids going through transplant in town, to say nothing of the adult patients. Taxi drivers, hotel managers, and restaurant waitstaff are accustomed to seeing seriously sick people coming and going in various stages of illness or convalescence. Here you could feel normal being abnormal.

Felicia ran into a middle-aged cancer patient from Texas at her hotel pool. He had a peach-sized tumor on his neck and a Powerball-winner smile on his face. Durham was his Lourdes. When Felicia told him why she'd come, his eyes lit up as he exclaimed, "You're in for a treat!"

The fateful meeting with Kurtzberg took place not on the upper floor of a towering medical center nor in the antiseptic chambers of a research lab, but in a modest, stand-alone brick building nestled among elm trees on Morreene Road, a side street a mile away from the main Duke University Hospital campus. Were it not for the signage one might mistake it for an insurance brokerage or a small local lawyer's office, but the humdrum exterior belies the drama that plays out inside. The offices of the Duke Pediatric Blood and Marrow Transplant Program have been a destination of last resort for families from all over the world. Some have arrived with shaky insurance coverage and literally pushed babies across its conference table, imploring the doctors to save their children's lives.

Kurtzberg managed the individual transplants herself for decades; now she was focused on research, though she retained the all-important duty of matching donor units to patients. The clinical supervision of the patients was now handled by a team led by Dr. Vinod Prasad, a tranquil, mustachioed virtuoso transplanter who'd been directly or indirectly involved in three thousand such procedures. He joined Kurtzberg at this initial meeting and would soon become one of the most important people in our lives.

Prasad began his career studying pediatrics in New Delhi. For someone interested in treating infectious disease in children, a large Indian hospital is what a South Side Chicago trauma center would be for a specialist in gunshot wounds. Prasad honed his craft in a place where twenty kids were admitted with meningitis *every day*. He grew so skilled he was able to diagnose some infections simply by smell. He'd later moved to London but landed at Duke after he fell in love with the bold, almost rock and roll attitude endemic to American medicine.

"In Europe a leukemia patient with multiple relapses gets sent to hospice care. In the United States the same patient gets sent into transplant," he once told me. "It's remarkable."

Kurtzberg had good news. "We've identified an excellent donor unit," she told Felicia. "If you agree to start the pre-transplant procedures immediately, we can admit him in three weeks."

Felicia was startled—after hearing repeatedly from Malech at the NIH that time was no issue, this sense of urgency was alarming. "W-why do you want to move so fast?"

"As a rule, we want to get the child to transplant as soon as possible because of the ongoing risk of something life-threatening," the doctor replied. "That would make a successful outcome harder to achieve. No one can predict when a child will get sick. It's like playing roulette."

Felicia was impressed with Kurtzberg's supreme confidence, but she was not ready to move forward yet. "When she and Sebastian left I felt like she was going to need some time," Kurtzberg recalled. "And I don't blame her. We've gotten pretty good at it, but transplant is still scary, risky, and not always successful."

Her qualms about timing aside, Felicia returned effulgent; you'd have thought she'd spent a week sipping mojitos and sunbathing in the Bahamas. At long last she'd found a path forward for us. Now all we had to do was find the courage to walk it.

A classic concept of twentieth-century psychology is the approach-avoidance conflict—the stressful ambivalence a decision-maker often feels when facing a goal with both advantages and disadvantages. Both forces tug at the decision-maker, and the avoidance urge strengthens as the goal gets closer.

Felicia and I knew transplant was the only sane option. But while Felicia was all in on Duke, I was still wary of picking a transplant center in a city where we had no family connections or built-in support system. The closer we came to the decision to go through with it, to really sit down and lay out a timetable, the more desperately I wanted to push it off.

We celebrated Sebastian's third birthday at the New York Transit Museum, a modest turnout of our friends and their kids frolicking through antique subway cars, a thick cake decorated with a cheery Thomas (of course) in blue frosting. The kid was in heaven. If only there were a repeat button to press at the end of your favorite days.

The next month we all headed to New Orleans for the biannual conference of the Immune Deficiency Foundation, the country's largest gathering of medical experts and patient families wrestling with the dozens of complex immune deficiencies nobody's ever heard of, CGD among them. Ostensibly we were there because Felicia was coming into her own as a patient advocate and had been invited to make some brief remarks during the CGD breakout session. On a deeper level, we were coming for assurance, an infusion of confidence that, yes, transplant was the way to go.

We reacquainted ourselves with many of the transplanters we'd met during our travels around the country, but the pivotal moment happened when we came face-to-face with a transplant survivor for the first time. His name was Rocco Fernandez, and with a radiant smile, which conveyed both boyhood wonder and ancient wisdom, he had the bearing of a bodhisattva. In many ways his family mirrored ours—Rocco was born with CGD, he had a rare HLA type due to the mixed ethnicity of his parents, and he'd undergone a cord blood transplant at Duke a few years back. His mother, Melissa, had been in touch with Felicia since shortly after our diagnosis and had sung the praises of Dr. Prasad and his "calming presence," so we were familiar with their story, but when we laid eyes on Rocco, cured and happy, reaching out to give Sebastian a hug, the emotion was overwhelming. Felicia and I turned away as the tears welled up.

"The power of community, as trite as it may sound, is critical," said John Boyle, the IDF president. "The isolation people feel, either literal or figurative, is a real problem, and one of the best remedies is meeting other people who are like you and hearing their stories." The conference can often feel like an extended pep rally, and rightfully so—treatment options are expanding so rapidly that almost every convention is a cavalcade of good news. Boyle insists he's not painting an overly rosy picture—according to their surveys 80 percent of immune deficiency patients have reported recent improvement in quality of life.

I was so moved by the hopeful vibe I volunteered to tell our story in the IDF video diary booth, discreetly editing out some of the more disgraceful episodes and trying to project my "natural nobility" as I stayed on message: with the right treatment and the right support, you don't have to let the condition crush you.

The stories of survival, endurance, and healing get the spotlight, but there are darker testimonies lurking in the hallways and the rear seats of the lobby bar—the adult patients going downhill, the parents who've lost a child. Some are mourning and have come to grieve and share; some are angry and have come to vent; a very few are truly unstable.

Those stories were haunting, but we would not be deterred. We returned from the convention resolved to pull the trigger and initiate the planning process with Duke. There were papers to be signed, insurance reps to consult, and medical workups not only for Sebastian but for Felicia and me as well.

Then, just as I was about to tell my bosses I needed to take time off and relocate, the approach-avoidance pendulum swung in the opposite direction.

Two bumps—"tumors" is the accurate medical term—appeared out of nowhere on Lydia's left knee. A pediatric oncologist said they were probably benign cysts, but to be sure she'd need minor surgery to have them removed and checked out by pathology.

Three anxiety-ravaged weeks later I walked Lydia back into another OR. Just as I'd done with Sebastian, I kissed her forehead as the anesthesiologist put her under, terrified that we'd have to confront another catastrophic diagnosis, this time with our precious daughter, the one pure, unimperiled presence in our lives.

The surgery was minor; waiting for the pathology results was major. For ten days the doomsday thinking chewed up my mind like a teaspoon that's slipped down a kitchen sink disposal. When we were finally summoned to the oncologist's office, they parked us in the waiting room for half an hour. It was the first time I'd been near kids undergoing chemo, and the looks on their quiet, masked faces were intense and penetrating. Their parents, attentive but drained, regarded us with the smiles of martyred saints. This was our future; the only question was whether one child would go through it or both.

"So, this turned out to be nothing," the oncologist began as he walked in. I don't recall anything else he said. I only remember looking at Felicia across the room and seeing her put her face into her hands. The minute the room cleared, we embraced and sobbed into each other's shoulders.

That little tango with pediatric oncology lasted barely a month. How would we survive a full calendar year of similar stresses with Sebastian? As the avoidance force kicked in we agreed to postpone the transplant till the following summer.

Avoidance had its advantages. That fall, we enrolled Sebastian in a local preschool. (Dr. Malech advises all parents, even those of healthy kids, to keep them out of school before age three; Sebastian was now old enough to get his doctor's blessing.) This was the first time he'd

ever spent any regular amount of time with other kids, and after growing jealous of his sister's daily departures to school, he was elated
that he could strap on a (Thomas the Tank Engine) backpack with purpose and kick off his academic career. "I get to go to school like sister!"
he exclaimed at drop-off. There were no first-day jitters—judging
from the smile in the photo we took, you'd think it was Christmas
morning.

His exultant spirits carried throughout the fall. Lydia's, however,
began trending down for the first time. I was at work one afternoon
when an email arrived from Felicia:

> [Lydia's second grade teacher] showed me a writing assign-
> ment where Lydia had drawn quite sad and moving pictures
> as well as words about how difficult it was to have a brother
> with CGD, with drawings of when he was born and people,
> such as the two of us crying in the hospital. Picture after pic-
> ture was like that. . . . I think Lydia has a lot of things to work
> through, and I suggested that she speak with the school psy-
> chologist.

It's common for the healthy sibling of a sick child to resent the extra
attention the sick kid gets. Felicia had done a great job preventing that
by scheduling special mommy-daughter days for shopping and one-
on-one dinners. But now Lydia, to date the most consistently upbeat
member of our family, was finally starting to show signs of the same
emotional gear grinding Felicia and I had been wrestling with for
three and a half years. We debated whether Lydia should come to North
Carolina at all. Perhaps, to spare her the trauma of seeing her brother
(and parents) going through that ordeal, it would be wiser to leave her
in Larchmont, under the care of my mom. Maybe it would be better if I
stayed too.

Prasad and Kurtzberg were steadfastly opposed. "We find that it's
better for the patient to have a sibling around. It helps on many levels."

That struck me as New Age woo-woo, but I let it drift. As for the fleeting thought that I'd stay behind? Kurtzberg was blunt. "Don't kid yourself. You want to be there for him." It was resolved: for better or worse we'd all be going.

We made it through that winter and arranged to spend spring break down at Duke, where I could meet the team, check out the hospital, and start exploring options for housing, work, and school.

We also knew that before we moved down there our marriage and our minds needed to be in sturdier conditions. The plan was to get a healthy dose of counseling, for us, and probably Lydia, to prep us for the ordeal.

Then the bottom fell out. Chaos made a comeback and the sorrows came, not single spies but in battalions.

My mom called. She'd gone to the emergency room with a case of appendicitis. The cause—a malignant tumor that had grown large enough to rupture through the tissue and enter her bloodstream. Major surgery and chemo were on the immediate horizon.

Felicia's mom called. She needed heart valve replacement surgery—they'd be opening her rib cage. The procedure would take place in Manhattan and she'd be staying with us during her recovery.

Then on March 14, Sebastian woke up in the middle of the night coughing. We took his temperature—a fever of 101. We gave him children's Tylenol and waited for one of two good things to happen—the abatement of those symptoms or the appearance of a runny nose. Neither occurred.

Thursday, March 17, as I watched the garbage men wistfully from my bedroom window, the cough was a low dry hack that came and went, subsiding just long enough to make us think we'd turned a corner, then returning, slow and unstoppable as Michael Myers in *Halloween*. The fever kept climbing. An ignoramus at a local hospital told us Sebastian had a run-of-the-mill cold—he thought CGD was an R&B

act. Felicia knew better: "My gut tells me something is not right," she reported. "I'm scared. Really scared."

Prasad told us to come down anyway. "If I'm going to do something in this situation, I want to be in charge. Whatever it is, we have what we need here to figure it out."

On Friday, the fever hit 104. Sebastian was trembling; for the first time there was fear in his eyes. Before he fell asleep he looked at Felicia and said, "Mom, I just want to be a normal boy." She promised him one day he would be.

On Saturday morning we were on the Delta flight that started this story. Sebastian's vomiting abated just as the plane landed. We hustled to Duke Children's Hospital in a rented minivan.

The main atrium was nearly deserted. As Sebastian coughed up the remaining contents of his stomach we wheeled his stroller to the elevators, ascended to the 24-hour walk-in clinic on the fourth floor, and buzzed in.

"We made it," Felicia said with hope in her eyes. *Yes*—I nodded in silent assent—*but have we made it in time . . . and will we ever make it back?*

Part 2

The Chimera Factory

March 2016–November 2016

Chapter 9

Q-tips

Please try to commit these instructions to memory. The life of your child depends on it.

Park across the street from the hospital. Stay at least six feet away from any other patients as you enter.

Sanitize your hands immediately using the Purell dispensers just inside the revolving doors.

Check in with the security guard if arriving after hours.

Walk to the main elevators. Do not press any buttons with your fingertips. Use a knuckle or an elbow.

Proceed to the fifth floor. Follow the signs to Unit 5200.

As you approach the main entrance to the Unit, do not touch the door handle. Press the blue call button and the desk nurse will buzz you into the antechamber. The exterior door will open if and only if the interior door is closed.

Once inside the antechamber, wait for the exterior door to close. Then perform the following actions in this exact sequence—place any nonessential personal items in your designated locker, wipe down every surface of any bags or luggage with the Clorox wipes on the

119

counter, cover your shoes with the paper booties, put on a face mask.
Then wash your hands thoroughly in the sink with the antibacterial
soap provided. DO NOT wash your hands until AFTER you've covered
your shoes.

Press the red door activator on the far wall and the interior door will
open (if and only if the exterior door is closed).

As you proceed to your child's room please pass by the nurses' station—
depending on the time of day there may be fresh results from the lab
you'll need to discuss.

Take a deep breath before you open the door. Whatever fear or sorrow
you're feeling, try to bury it—the patients pick up on anxiety.

Now—go in there and perform the one task none of the doctors or
nurses can: be a parent.

Sebastian was admitted to the Pediatric Blood and Marrow Transplant Unit—alternately called the PBMTU or Unit 5200—the day after we arrived in Durham. We'd planned to visit for five days. Sebastian wouldn't go home for eight months.

We'd spent much of the previous day camped in an examination room at the outpatient clinic of Duke Children's Hospital, formally known as the Valvano Day Hospital. (Jim Valvano, the NC State basketball coach and deceased cancer patient/fundraiser, became a legend in both collegiate sports and medical research.) Sebastian had no fever upon arrival but spiked a frightening 104.4 within two hours. The attending staff took his labs, put in an IV, and kept him on his current meds until they could schedule a CT scan for the next morning. The place was stocked with games and puzzles—I popped a Klonopin and settled in for an afternoon of Sorry! and Connect Four.

By 7 p.m. that evening they'd concluded he was "well appearing and active" enough to be discharged for the night. We took down the 24-hour emergency number and headed to the nearby Ronald McDonald House for the night.

The Ronald McDonald Houses (RMH) are among the most underappreciated blessings of American philanthropy. Tucked inconspicuously near large medical centers, they cumulatively house thousands of families with kids in need of long-term hospital care, sparing them the financial burden of months-long hotel stays or apartment rentals. The Durham RMH, just down Erwin Road from the main entrance to Duke Hospital, is a brick structure built somewhat like a mountain lodge. The large reception area opens into a living room with a fireplace where kids can play board games. A little Latino kid with no hair was purchasing Park Place as we entered, passing a life-size statue of Ronald himself holding a boy and accepting flowers from a little girl. We proceeded to complete the paperwork needed to get our room keys and red wristbands. Someone had called ahead and approved us; we were expected.

In a daze from the day's events, we listened to the receptionist run down the rules and policies. "A ten-dollar-per-night donation is suggested but not required. No pets are allowed. Smoking is permitted only in designated areas. And," he said, pointing to the relevant section of a written agreement, "we have a zero-tolerance policy on alcohol and drugs."

I scrawled my signature on the form and we got a quick tour. The house featured fifty-five guest rooms, a playground, a computer room, an outdoor grill, and a large common kitchen frequently abuzz with youth volunteers preparing meals for the guests. A shuttle bus left for the hospital every two hours. Thanks to the charity of the community, free passes were available to nearby museums and attractions.

Given Sebastian's condition, we were allotted one of the suites for the immunocompromised; it had its own kitchenette and laundry. Felicia dealt with Sebastian's meds and feeding as I schlepped in the luggage. She retreated with him into the bedroom for the night, while I lay down on the couch. It was the first week of the NCAA basketball tournament, and as this was North Carolina I figured, when in Rome. Flicking on the TV, I tried to get into an early-round David-Goliath matchup that had quickly become a ritual slaughter, but swan-dived into sleep before the first Geico ad.

We breakfasted the next morning in the big kitchen and dining hall with other families who'd availed themselves of the donated groceries in the permanently stocked fridge and pantry. The place had the same eerie quiet of a doctor's waiting room, as if everyone's situation was so precarious a single loud voice might trigger a code blue. We swallowed a few spoonfuls of yogurt and oatmeal and hurried back to the hospital for the CT scan.

While I typically accompanied the kids into surgery, Felicia oversaw radiology procedures—a tougher gig, since the kids stay awake and need to hold still. "Mommy's going to take you to the Giant Donut and make sure everything is okay," she assured Sebastian in her sweet baby voice, deploying one of many cute, kid-friendly names for medical devices and procedures she'd neologized to keep him at ease.

In the maw of the imposing machine, it was harder for him to keep cool. As he often did when he was nervous, he reverted to his preverbal *grrrr* and *hmmmmrr* sounds to convey his emotions.

"The Giant Donut doesn't hurt," Felicia explained, "it takes pictures of the inside of your body. You just need to be really, really still—like a statue—so the donut doctor can get a good picture. You can do that, right, my baby?"

Sebastian held Felicia closely. He wanted his mother to take him away from this: to go home and play trains and be "all better." Soon, however, a familiar look of determination came upon his features and he said, "Okay, Mommy."

Felicia laid him gingerly on the molded plastic cradle. Sebastian assumed the countenance and pose of the statue on Henry V's sarcophagus. Felicia stood beside him in her lead apron, watching the dark hole swallow her child.

Thanks to those assiduous efforts, the machine rewarded us with a large, legible image of our worst fears.

On the radiograph, our son's little lungs looked like they'd been decorated with that cottony store-bought spider webbing with which suburbanites decorate front-yard shrubbery on Halloween. The wispy strands were spangled with little white nodules resembling the heads of Q-tips. Dozens of them.

"The wheels are coming off" was the candid professional assessment of Dr. Paul Martin, the PBMTU's answer to Jeff Bridges: tall, mellow, and gifted with a knack for giving hard-core news with a tone of casual tranquility. Earlier in his career he'd even sported a ponytail.

Martin's message was clear—the scaffolding of preventative measures we'd constructed to prop up Sebastian's health was collapsing. The Q-tips meant his lungs were under attack; the situation was urgent. If the problem wasn't arrested, he could die. The cherry on top— as we took off Sebastian's little shoes and socks, I noticed a red swollen mass on the bottom of his right heel—a new abscess in a new spot. His whole system was crashing. "Due to the complexity of care needed," read the antiseptic language of the medical records, "it was determined that the patient would need to be managed inpatient."

As we wheeled Sebastian from the Valvano Day Hospital to Unit 5200, a familiar feeling engulfed us—the bear hug of admission into another labyrinthine children's hospital. Once again, we were crossing the threshold into Hospitalworld from a place where we had control over our decisions and our time to a place where that control was surrendered almost entirely to others. The hermetically sealed sanctum of the Unit—a hospital within a hospital—squared the effect. I harkened back to a lesson from the meditation teaching, decreed so casually in books and seminars: the spirit can get bigger when the ego gets smaller. This would be a prime opportunity to road test that claim.

To say the patient rooms on the Unit are small is like saying Orson Welles put on a few pounds in his later years. Empty, it would feel like a midtown Manhattan hotel room; subtract the floor space occupied by the bed and medical equipment, it's closer to a cell in San Quentin. Cram the clothing in a corner; stow the toys under the bed. A cushioned bench built into the far wall suffices as a couch by day, a caregiver sleeping space at night. Anyone taller than five foot three will be sleeping in the fetal position.

Since it was clear Sebastian was sick, but unclear what exactly he was sick *with*, we got the deluxe treatment. His presence on the Unit made him (and us) a danger to the other patients, most of whom were profoundly immunocompromised either by their original disease or from the transplant itself. (One of the top priorities of any transplant unit is ensuring that the patients don't infect each other, which is why each room has its own self-contained HEPA filter system.) Consequently, Sebastian was confined to his room at all times. Any nurses or doctors who came in first donned surgical scrubs and masks as well as the usual gloves. The look is not quite as hard-core as the outfits you see in footage from Ebola hot zones or COVID-19 drive-through testing centers, but from the patient's perspective it still looks like a crew of yellow spacemen have invaded your bedroom. Charming.

Scarier for us was the uncertainty. Once again it was medical mystery hour. The Q-tips in the lungs had been located, but nobody knew quite what was causing them. Without a trustworthy diagnosis, there could be no trustworthy treatment plan.

The most likely explanation was bacterial infection. The top candidates were *Klebsiella*, *Burkholderia*, *Nocardia*, *Serratia*, and *Pseudomonas*. (For some reason the names of many bacteria sound like science-fiction villainesses.) If it was a fungal infection, *Aspergillus* was the prime suspect.

"Where do you think he might have been infected?" I asked Felicia during Sebastian's nap time. The question was nitroglycerine, an open invitation to play the blame game, but as previously stated, medical matters were our default conversation topic.

"It could have been anywhere—probably the preschool. I know they send out notices whenever a kid comes down with anything, but the kids spend half the day sharing toys and touching each other. We accepted that risk when we agreed to send him to school."

"Yeah, well, we didn't want to keep him locked up forever." We both took that safe off-ramp from the conversation and went back to our respective phone screens. In my head, however, I was replaying a moment from two weeks earlier when I'd been playing hide-and-seek with the kids at a local playground. While I was It, Sebastian had hidden in a space under one of the slides. Finding him there on his stomach among the wood chips and dirt, I'd gasped and whisked him away. Petrified I'd endangered him by letting my guard down, I'd kept the incident a secret from Felicia. Unbeknownst to me, she was harboring her own secret fear—that he'd contracted the infection a few weeks earlier when she'd let him play for a few minutes in a friend's garden.

Focused on our silent self-flagellation, we'd ignored another possibility—an odd scenario particular to CGD patients. The immune system, as previously stated, is a team of different cells, each with a different function. In CGD patients, the neutrophils don't work, but the rest of the system frequently tries to compensate by maintaining a state of upregulation. This can lead the body, with the smallest provocation, to go into overdrive and cause an inordinate inflammatory response. Curiously, that alone can lead to an elevated white blood cell count and formulation of granulomas—clumps of white blood cells—in the lungs, *even if there is no significant underlying infection*. A high fever and cough, the identical symptoms of infection, often appear with this peculiar inflammatory response as well—once again, the quirks of a rare immune deficiency hiding behind common symptoms. "It's a strange disease," says Prasad.

As Sebastian unpacked some of his beloved trains and got his umpteenth IV, this was the riddle: bona fide infection or just inflammation? The difference between a right and wrong answer could mean the difference between life or death. Standard treatment for granulomas caused by inflammation is a heavy dose of steroids—anti-inflammatories that inhibit the immune system. If you botch the diagnosis and prescribe steroids when the issue *isn't* inflammation at all, but a raging fungal infection, you are blocking the body's only way of fighting that infection and letting it run wild—essentially, adding gasoline to a fire. Conversely, if you treat inflammation with antibiotics, you'll be letting the granulomas grow uninhibited. If they get big enough, eventually they can block an artery or choke off an organ. If your goal is to kill the patient, these misdiagnoses are slow but effective ways to do it.

Nailing this diagnosis would be a conundrum. Absolute certainty required a lung biopsy, which in Sebastian's case would mean another surgery under sedation, the insertion of a needle through his ribs in the back, the extraction of tissue, and the risk of hemorrhaging, infection, or lung collapse. (In this branch of medicine, procedures and treatments are often as dangerous as the diseases they're meant to address.)

It was Sunday, and Martin and the other doctors wanted to get the sign-off from Prasad before they took that drastic step. Wagering on infection, they started an augmented regimen of IV antibiotics and awaited Prasad's return the next morning.

This was all happening during a turning point in Sebastian's cognitive development. He was weeks away from his fourth birthday, roughly the age when the brain first becomes capable of forming long-term memories and when a child patient can verbalize his or her internal feelings accurately enough to be able to assist in his/her own care. (This was one of the reasons Malech had recommended waiting till age four for transplant.) I recently asked Sebastian what he remembers about entering the Unit for the first time. "I was scared," he answered, "because I thought I was going to get lots of shots. And . . . divorce."

Despite his age, Sebastian was sufficiently perspicacious to realize his condition had become the root cause of much of our domestic discord. He feared what this visit to Hospitalworld might do to his family as much as what it could do to his body. But in fact, despite the terror of the immediate situation, Felicia and I were deeply relieved—we'd come to the right place; we'd shut out all the other distractions; we could finally focus on this process and see it through as a team.

Knowing they'd be in that room indefinitely I left to pick up some food and retrieve some toiletries. As I left the Unit for the first time and took the paper booties off my shoes, I exhaled four years' worth of anticipatory stress. "That's that," I said in a tone that would have tickled the high priests of radical acceptance. "The doctors have him now."

Prasad made his entrance the next day, serene and confident as Vishnu the Preserver. It was the first time I'd been in his physical presence, and I felt the air around him vibrate. He was everything I was not—regally composed, supremely accomplished, and endowed with a compassion commensurate with his competence. Had I not been so grateful to see him I would have been writhing with jealousy.

Prasad still didn't know what was wrong with our son, but whatever it was, he knew he could deal with it. Aside from the pediatric hellscapes he'd traversed back in New Delhi, he'd wrestled with some of the world's most formidable CGD cases of the past twenty years and emerged victorious. "When I first came to Duke, we had a patient who presented with what looked like a golf ball on the side of his chest," he told me. "It was a fungal lung infection that had grown so massive it was protruding out of the rib cage."

"Wha . . . what's the treatment for *that?*"

"We ordered a major lung resection and eliminated enough of the infection to send the kid into transplant," he said matter-of-factly. His placid scientific manner notwithstanding, this man was a rock and roll transplanter ready to go balls to the wall if need be.

In Sebastian's case, Prasad could afford to tread more cautiously. He didn't want to order a lung biopsy before he'd tried everything else. The next step would be a bronchoscopy—the insertion of a tube down the throat—to see what cultures might be retrievable. During that procedure, while Sebastian was under, they'd also insert something called a PICC line (peripherally inserted central catheter) so they could give Sebastian medicine and nutrition and draw blood without having to stick him as much.

Prasad was already thinking further down the road. We were origi-nally planning to move down to Durham after the school year ended and go into transplant in July. That timetable was now deep-sixed. "It makes no sense to wait," Prasad said, gesticulating with the arm of his glasses like a conductor's baton for emphasis. "As soon as he's healthy enough, we need to go." In fact, Prasad had already ordered the final round of HLA blood typing to identify the best donor match in the cord blood bank.

In medical terms, the path ahead was straightforward—clear the lungs, find the match, go into transplant. In practical terms, things were considerably more complex—find a school for Lydia where she could transfer ASAP, find out what to do about my job, find a place to stay down in Durham, figure out what would happen with our house back in New York. In psychological terms, the accelerated timeline came as a shock—we thought we'd have months to get ready for this emotionally. Instead it would play out as the classic nightmare where you show up to calculus class wholly unprepared for that morning's AP exam.

We'd brought Lydia with us to the Unit that morning, but there are strict rules governing sibling visits and she was not allowed in. Prasad explained there was a particularly virulent strain of the flu going around Durham that spring, and they didn't want to risk her presence in case she was carrying it. I had to park her on the hallway floor outside the door to the antechamber.

Literally within three hours of Prasad's warning, Lydia said she felt hot. Her temperature hit 102. Accompanying flu symptoms arrived shortly thereafter. Neither she nor I could go on the Unit while she was contagious, nor could we be in any of the public spaces at the Ronald McDonald House. We quarantined ourselves in our room with medicine, TV, and takeout pizza, which she threw up that night. The next day the same bug turned me into a quivering mess under the bedsheets. It was a harrowing week.

Back on the Unit, Felicia was in the belly of the beast, cut off from the outside world and unable to tag-team with me for a break. Sebastian's fever finally subsided, but the mystery of the Q-tips had yet to resolve and for some reason his red blood cell count was also dropping; he wasn't getting enough iron. His face was pale, his body flaccid. Compounding the stress, Felicia's mom was undergoing heart valve replacement surgery that same week—the procedure required a bone saw. She'd come to New York so Felicia could be there to help her recover. Now Felicia was marooned in North Carolina and might not be back for a year. Helpless, Felicia let it all go at night after Sebastian went down. "I cried helplessly, with massive, uncontrollable tears," she recalled, "like the weak and terrified lonely person I was."

Weak and terrified, yes. But she was not, in fact, alone. Her son was there, and despite his age and condition he was able to offer support.

After the initial shock of the first few days in the Unit wore off, Sebastian adjusted to his new environment and began to appreciate its single silver lining—he had Mommy all to himself. No sister, no housework, no work calls to partition her attention. As his spirits lifted, he sustained his mother through those first frightening days.

By the end of the week something remarkable had happened—out of nowhere, a group of people who had never met Sebastian emerged semi-spontaneously to encircle our crisis and warm us in the embrace of the Duke community. Preparing for the visit, I'd reached out to an old friend named Tina Merrill—a woman with whom I'd been tight in high school and college but hadn't seen in years. As I let the friendship atrophy she'd gotten married, had a son, and moved to Durham, where she worked as the CFO of a local tech company. I'd figured she was neck-deep in her own life and wouldn't be able to do much other than give some tips on schools and restaurants. Instead, she volunteered to essentially drop everything to help us. Primarily that meant assisting with Lydia, who was instantly adopted into Tina's family.

Felicia also reconnected with a childhood friend from Chicago, Jessica Yang, who happened to be in nursing school at Duke. Just as Tina did with me, Jessica responded immediately when Felicia reached out through Facebook, and offered to help us with our mounting logistical needs—car seats, clothing, and so on. "It was not a burden, it was a joy," Jessica says. "To me this was just an extension of what nursing care is: to be present, to offer support."

We would soon see that the nurses on the Unit felt the same way. Many of them choose to work there specifically because they value the deep and intense emotional bonds they form with patients and their families. For medical professionals who value human contact, the intimacy of the Unit is much preferred over the conveyor belt atmosphere of an OR or ER.

There are about twenty assigned to the Unit at any given time. Each has an opportunity to volunteer to be part of the primary team for each patient. That first week, a relatively new nurse named Liz Vaughn stepped forward to be one of Sebastian's primaries. "I just love that age," she told us. "Three-, four-, five-year-old boys. They're hilarious; and they know what's going on, but not enough for it to really dampen their day-to-day mood. They just go with it." Over the course of the coming months, as she guided Sebastian through his time on the Unit, we would witness a degree of giving and care—what author Larissa MacFarquhar describes as "superaltruism"—that I'd only heard about on heartstring-tugger evening news end pieces.

The nurses were supplemented by a steady stream of volunteers, many of them Duke premed undergrads who came to play with Sebastian for a few hours so Felicia could escape the Unit for a short walk or a bite at the cafeteria. Others were laity from local churches. Then there was Tray the music guy, who'd swing through a couple of times a week with his guitar and harmonica. Cumulatively, they formed a makeshift army of the kind.

Felicia also found support from the other patient families. One in particular was a pleasant surprise—just down the hall, Felicia saw the name Thor over one of the patient doors. It was baby Thor Richels from Minnesota and his parents, Justine and Scott, whom we'd met at the immune deficiency conference the year before in New Orleans. At the time, guided by their immunologist, they weren't even considering transplant. The conference, numerous follow-up conversations with Felicia, and their subsequent research had changed their minds. Without telling us, they'd come here a month before, and Thor, just eighteen months old, was sailing through the process. Their broad, Minnesota-nice smiles were a welcome counterbalance to the funereal silence that often hung on the hallway.

"So . . . you decided to go through with the transplant?" Felicia asked incredulously after an initial hug and hello.

"Oh, yaah," said Justine. "We just did more research and decided to do it. Plus, we got pregnant again and when we tested Layla in utero it turned out she was a match for Thor. So, I just gave birth to her here and we're using her cord blood as a donor." The Richelses had a wild setup—a newborn back at the Ronald McDonald House and a transplant kid on the Unit. If they could manage this, so could we.

These are the kind of folks one might expect to meet, but fate also dealt us a wild card—a semi-famous private investigator named Hunter Glass. I'd anticipated that my boss would put me in charge of any stories originating out of the Carolinas while I was there, and as it happens my show had just initiated production on a local cold-case murder Hunter had been working. I took him to lunch that first week, if for no other reason than to put a cheeseburger on the expense account and my mind on anything other than infectious disease.

Within minutes I recognized Hunter as one of those colorful Southern-fried characters who seems to have just escaped from the pages of a *True Detective* script. A veteran of the 82nd Airborne and a retired gang unit cop, he's the kind of politically incorrect crime fighter who'd refer to Chewbacca as a "house Wookiee." There were a half-dozen reasons for his red state sensibility to clash with my northeastern college boy shtick. Instead, we hit it off. "You might be a dick," he said after sizing me up, "but I think you're my kind of dick." We spent a good hour talking about the details of his case, but he was probing for cracks and soon got me to reveal the real reason I was in town.

Hunter takes the Southern hospitality thing as seriously as the Pledge of Allegiance, and immediately volunteered to help. A place to crash, a car to borrow, help with the local cops, weapons—he was happy to provide all of the above. "I've seen situations like this destroy families," he said as I headed back to the hospital. "Let's not let that happen."

As this local support system coalesced, we got some good news on the medical front. For reasons no one could explain, Sebastian's red blood cell count turned around just hours before a required transfusion—a bit of good news that earned a place in Felicia's catalogue of miracles.

Sebastian's procedure yielded more good news—his PICC line went in without incident and the culture from the bronchoscopy tested positive for small amounts of the bacteria *Pseudomonas*. That datum and the abatement of fever led some of the Duke doctors to conclude the puzzle of the Q-tips had been solved. The inflammation/infection mystery was resolved in favor of infection, they claimed, and the treatment could proceed as such.

Up at NIH, Dr. Malech, who'd been monitoring the situation daily—wasn't as sure. *Pseudomonas* tends to be something that can cause infections in the elderly or in diabetics, he reasoned, but it did not make sense in the specific context of a young child with CGD. Those doubts notwithstanding, the plan was to proceed with the current infection-targeted treatment for two weeks, then take another CT scan.

In the meantime, Sebastian had tested negative for a slate of other pathogens—now that they'd been ruled out he could leave his room and roam about the Unit. There was a tricycle in the storage closet, and he soon made it his business to pedal laps up and down the hall of the L-shaped unit like Danny on his Big Wheel in *The Shining*. Prasad thought he could be discharged to the Ronald McDonald House in a few days and complete the rest of the pre-transplant treatment as an outpatient.

By week's end Lydia and I were healthy enough to visit Carolina Friends, a Quaker school where Tina sent her son, Sam. The school was one of those hippie-trippy "big hug" places that eschewed testing and bragged about its gender-neutral bathrooms (a hot-button issue in the Tar Heel state at the time). Kids started each day with a "settling-in session" to center themselves; they were introduced to Spanish during art class; they learned biology in mud boots while hunting tadpoles in the campus creek. It wasn't how I was taught, but it was precisely what our daughter needed—a nurturing environment where she could find community and love during a time of upheaval. Box checked. One less thing to worry about.

We headed to Tina's house for dinner that night as Felicia and Sebastian remained on lockdown on the Unit. Tina's husband, Dave, genuinely trying to comfort a man he'd barely met, offered me a glass of bourbon, but I was still so ill I couldn't imagine drinking. "Take the bottle," he implored. "Put it to use when you feel better."

I had to head back to New York with Lydia and cobble together a plan to move us down to Durham within the coming weeks. I arranged with the RMH to keep our room even though it would be vacant for the two days after we left and before Felicia and Sebastian arrived. I made sure the sheets were laundered so they wouldn't catch our flu and stocked the fridge with groceries. After swinging by the Unit to say goodbye and drop off the rental car, I grabbed Lydia and the bags and headed to the airport with Hunter at the wheel of his black Mercury Marauder. I was satisfied we'd made it through a grueling week with both our son and our marriage in stable condition and a clear action plan moving forward. Felicia's stamina and focus had her on the road to sainthood; and as for myself, at least I'd done what I'd been told. Crucially, I hadn't made things worse. Or so I thought.

"Sometimes I can't stand you! I just can't STAAAND YOU!!!!"

This was Felicia calling me from the Ronald McDonald House. In a narrative adorned with epithets, she explained what had happened.

After I'd departed, the RMH housekeeping staff had entered the room to sanitize every surface. While doing so they discovered the bottle of bourbon I'd accepted from Tina's husband and absentmindedly left behind. The staff immediately alerted management.

Now the day manager was on the phone.

"Sir, the alcohol found in your room constitutes a clear violation of our zero-tolerance policy, which you signed the night you arrived."

"I thought that meant I couldn't be intoxicated while staying there, and I wasn't."

"No alcohol is allowed on the premises, sir."

"What's zero tolerance mean?"

"I'm afraid it means immediate expulsion from the property."

"Okay. . . . Well . . . I've already left."

"The policy applies to the entire family, including the patient."

"What? For how long?"

"Permanently."

My excuses came spewing forth like rounds from a minigun. *It wasn't my bottle; it was just a present from a friend I accepted to be a good guest; I've been sick, it would have been impossible for me to drink.* As I uttered the words I realized how they sounded precisely like the yammering denials of a problem drinker. They bounced harmlessly off the bureaucrat's hide.

It didn't matter that I, the offending party, was off the premises and four hundred miles north; it didn't matter that Sebastian's health was hanging in the balance; nor did it matter that Felicia was now responsible for administering regular doses of medicine through his PICC line by herself and keeping it sterile. Tha rules was tha rules, and there was no room for appeal.

With scalding shame rising from my collar, I fumbled for a fix. "Oh God, oh God, *oh God, oh GOD!*" I blurted into the phone. Could we move into a hotel? Tina's house? Hunter's? I could smell my wife's scorn coming through the phone. I'd managed to make a hideous mess and I had no workable solution.

Mercifully, Duke did. As Felicia called the hospital, pleading for help, a family coordinator told us about a remarkable nonprofit called

Hayden's Journey of Inspiration (HJI) that provides long-term housing specifically for families undergoing stem cell transplant at Duke. The foundation is named after a young leukemia patient successfully transplanted at Duke in 2004–2005. Since then, her family has raised funds to purchase, maintain, and furnish three large units in a nearby apartment complex that qualified families can occupy for as long as necessary, rent free. Just as we were getting the big red boot from Ronald McDonald, a vacancy was opening up. Salvation.

Days later, as Felicia was moving into the apartment with Tina's and Jessica's help, Prasad, Kurtzberg, and the doctors on the Unit were assembled at a staff meeting. On Mondays the agenda typically involves updating the team on anything of note that's transpired over the weekend with current patients. Then the discussion turns to patients in the pre-transplant phase. Have they found a good matched unit? When would they come? Has their insurance cleared? Have they sorted out housing?

Kurtzberg had an important update on Sebastian—she'd found a match. And not just any match—a beautiful five out of six HLA match, nearly perfect. On top of that, this donor unit's cell dose was high—given Sebastian's weight there would be more than enough to engraft successfully.

Felicia was required to bring Sebastian to the day clinic for regular blood tests; and on her next visit Prasad ran to tell her the news: as soon as Sebastian's lungs cleared, we could go into transplant. Our quest was over—*WE HAD A MATCH!*

Trouble was, the lungs weren't clearing. The antibiotic regimen kicked back most of Sebastian's symptoms, but the next CT scan showed only mild improvement in the size and number of the Q-tip nodules. Unless we wanted to do a lung biopsy, we'd have to continue in this holding pattern, taking the same medications for two more weeks and then taking another look. This was our first lesson in "patience with patients"—once you've embarked on the transplant process, waiting an extra two weeks, or even two months for an infection to clear is par for the course. At the time of this writing the family living in our old HJI apartment has been stranded in limbo for a full calendar year waiting for their daughter to get over a nasty virus and its related complications. Hospitalworld runs on its own clock.

Felicia had support from Tina, Jessica, and cousins who flew in from out of state to lend a hand for a few days, but she spent most of her time alone with Sebastian. As they acclimated to the apartment, she tried to explain what was going on and what was to come, using his beloved Thomas the Tank Engine as an educational aid. "We know that Thomas sometimes needs a battery transplant so he can feel better and do what he wants to do," she cooed. "And Sebastian is also going to get a transplant—with some new supercells in his body so he can go back to school and won't need any more medicine." She drew a series of pictures showing the old yucky cells getting sucked out of his cartoon body and new, smiling cells taking their place. The last frame depicted a healthy Sebastian jumping into his parents' arms.

He indicated some level of understanding. If he was scared he didn't show it.

In New York two weeks later, our Subaru was laden with suitcases and boxes as Lydia and I pulled out of the driveway and began the drive down to Durham. Felicia's mom, attended by a visiting nurse and some warmhearted neighbors, was en route to a full recovery and would soon be well enough to head home. Lydia and I cranked the radio and told stories all the way down. Despite the dire circumstances, we knew we were about to be reunited as a family and begin one of the most important and transformative experiences of our lives. Whatever we were doing, we were finally *moving forward.*

When we pulled into the parking lot outside the HJI apartment the following afternoon, I felt like I'd been there before, on business. The property is part of Alden Place, one of those sprawling town house complexes that have become a bedrock of the rental housing market in twenty-first-century America. Many a newsworthy crime takes place in similar environs, which is why it looked so familiar to me, but the amenities were impressive—two swimming pools and exercise rooms, common grill areas, and even a little car wash. Given our RMH experience, I was stunned at our good fortune.

The three HJI apartments are all in one building. Ours was on the ground floor—a sliding door in the living room opened out onto a small patio facing the parking lot. Felicia gave me a cautious reception, and after we unpacked the Outback the four of us went out to grab a slice at Sebastian's new favorite pizza place. We were asleep by eight.

The following morning was Lydia's first day at Carolina Friends. We all piled into the rental car to drop her off as she joined her classmates for some Quaker-based education in the Mountain Room. On the woodsy ten-minute drive back Felicia and I talked through our new status as a two-car family: she'd keep the rental to take to Sebastian's appointments that day, while I'd drive the Outback to the local affiliate, where I'd been assigned a spare office.

"Uh . . . where's the Subaru?" I asked as we pulled up to the apartment. The Outback had been parked in front when we left; now it was gone. We rushed into the apartment to try to make sense of things and spotted two clues within seconds: the patio door was open, and Felicia's purse was missing. I suddenly recalled hearing a rustling noise during the night. I'd gotten out of bed to investigate, seen the patio door open, and assumed the sound was just the wind blowing the blinds against it. Surely no one would burgle the home of a transplant patient?

Yes, they would. After we called the cops, the patrol officer who rolled up told us it's quite common for thieves to case complexes like Alden Place and break into ground-floor units if they can open the patio door. We'd graciously left the door open, of course. Someone had noticed, entered while we were sleeping, snatched Felicia's purse, then waited for us to leave the next morning to use her key to drive off with our car.

Felicia was shaking. There's a unique feeling of violation that accompanies any home invasion, but what made this extra creepy was the knowledge that they'd been watching us less than an hour earlier as we left with our kids for school. Would these people come back? Did they know we were uniquely vulnerable with a sick child? Could we ever feel safe in this apartment again?

This is bad. Don't make it worse. Breathe . . . and detach. I resolved to make this moment a time to shine. All the counseling, the meditation, the medication—my Program—was crafted for situations such as this. Fighting the pull of anger, panic, and blame, I refused to let a mindless reaction strip me of my natural nobility this time.

"A car like this, I wouldn't figure to wind up in a chop shop like a Ferrari or a Lambo," explained the responding officer. "Gangbangers prolly just took it for a joyride. Good chance we find it abandoned in the next couple of days." After giving him the car's make and plate number, I calmly thanked him for his help. We exchanged cell numbers. Twenty minutes later a chubby college kid arrived in an orange Kia Soul and Ubered me to work.

That afternoon I got a call—the Outback had turned up in a skeevy part of East Durham. The cops thought it might have been used for a drive-by and ditched. My iPod and the laptop Felicia had in her purse were long gone, but I was welcome to come pick up the car if I wanted to avoid a towing charge.

I retrieved the Outback. I had it detailed to rid the interior of lingering menthol cigarette stink. Surrendering to the chaos, I drove it back to the apartment, the place we'd be calling home until the doctors said we could have our lives back. My wife and I hugged. For the time being, at least, I was done fucking up.

Chapter 10

Please Sign Here

....

"Yes, it's scary," Dr. Prasad said flatly. "It's supposed to be scary."

The "it" in question was the nine-page Pediatric Treatment Plan he'd fanned out in front of us across the conference table at the PBMTU office on Morreene Road. The meeting had the mechanics of a real estate closing—documents, disclosures, dotted lines. Felicia and I sat nervously in our chairs, shifting weight from bun to bun, as Sebastian played in the corner, sorting out issues of roundhouse etiquette with his trains. He'd been there for a solid hour while Prasad walked through every step of the transplant road map in excruciating detail.

Stem cell transplantation had been outlined to us several times already. This time was different. We were now just days away from admission to the Unit and Duke required us to acknowledge that we'd been informed of every possible problem we could encounter along the way. There was a signature line on each page.

Every American television viewer is familiar with the format of the sixty-second pharmaceutical ad. They all begin with a middle-aged consumer testifying to the miraculous benefits of some new drug, overlaid with images of said consumer engaged in a blissful everyday activity formerly forbidden by their condition (picking up the grandkids, wearing sleeveless dresses, exchanging precoital glances with a partner). Scenes from the felicitously restored lifestyle continue over the final twenty seconds of the spot while a speed-reading announcer sprints through the potential side effects.

The hypothetical ad for a stem cell transplant would be ten minutes long, the final nine reserved for the adverse reaction rundown.

Known side effects include:

Mouth sores; rash; alopecia (hair loss); weakness; somnolence; peripheral neuropathy; low platelet counts that can lead to bleeding complications in the digestive tract and bladder; pulmonary toxicity; fever; congestion; vomiting; diarrhea; seizures; abnormal liver function; water retention; weakening of the heart muscle; bloody urine; bad taste in the mouth; stomach pain; headaches; pain in the joints; breakdown in the red blood cells; hives; difficulty breathing; bone pain; enlargement of the spleen; allergic reaction; potential fatal bleeding in the brain; blood vessel injury; nerve injury; clotting; infection; bone marrow depression; fluid overload; infection from every known pathogen, including hepatitis, CMV, and HIV; acute or chronic GvHD; interstitial pneumonia; organ damage; developmental and cognitive impairment. And of course, cancer.

The consent form spelled out each of these with clinical precision. For those parents who needed reminding, it explicitly stated that in some cases these side effects "are potentially dangerous, life-threatening, or fatal." And with a stylistic flourish only a lawyer could summon, the document cloaked itself with a universal disclaimer: "There may be additional side effects that are not known or predictable at this time."

Tucked into all that text was an additional waiver that came as a true surprise—to proceed we had to acknowledge that this cord blood transplant was not—repeat, *not*—an FDA-approved procedure. The FDA had approved Duke's cord blood procedure in 2012, but our donor unit had been collected and stored at the Carolinas Cord Blood Bank before then. A confidence booster, it wasn't.

"My God," I gasped. "I know you have to disclose all this, but realistically, what are his chances of making it?"

Prasad took off his glasses and used them to poke the air. "I can tell you this. Every patient gets *some* of these side effects; nobody gets *all* of them." It was clear he'd used that line before.

"So . . . ?"

"Ninety percent. Ninety percent chance he makes it."

"And a ten percent chance he dies."

"I believe your math is correct."

Prasad says some parents arrive at Duke determined to transplant, only to flip at the last minute; with others the reverse occurs. Felicia and I looked over at Sebastian, took a deep breath, and signed. This was not just a fatalistic surrender to the inevitable. In the past weeks we'd seen Prasad make a daring call—a William Tell shot that required as much nerve as skill. It played out perfectly. He'd aced his audition.

Here's what happened. As previously noted, the Q-tip nodules on Sebastian's lungs hadn't disappeared. In fact, a CT scan taken the week after our apartment was burgled showed them increasing. We were devastated.

Boldly disregarding the skepticism of some of his colleagues, Prasad did a one-eighty. On April 21 he ordered a colonoscopy on a hunch the initial diagnosis of infection had been wrong all along. He now believed the problem was inflammation. If he was right, there'd likely be granulomas in the gut as well as the lungs.

The scope found precisely that. Prasad fearlessly flipped Sebastian's treatment, cutting back the antibiotic and putting him on a regimen of strong steroids. If the inflammation thesis was right, the lungs would clear in a few more weeks. If it was wrong, if the granulomas in the intestine were a separate problem and the lungs were beset by persistent infection as first suspected, catastrophe loomed.

While we waited to see if the doctor's wager paid off, the pre-transplant workup continued apace. The team proceeded to test every testable part of Sebastian's body, making sure he was infection free and hearty enough to withstand the coming onslaught of the transplant. They needed him in top form to withstand the pending annihilation of his existing immune system. If there was any lingering or suppressed infection hiding anywhere in the body, it could then run rampant, with fatal consequences. Of the many ironies and inversions of this brave new Hospitalworld, one of the most bizarre was that the doctors strained to get their patients as healthy as possible *before* admission, and then, in the confines of the Unit, lovingly brought them to the brink of death.

For weeks, after breakfast and morning meds, Daddy left with Lydia bound for school and office, while Mommy and Sebastian headed to the hospital, where he was prepped like a prospective astronaut prior to a space mission. Lab tests for dozens of viruses—herpes simplex, Epstein-Barr virus, CMV, vancomycin-resistant enterococcus. Scans of the kidney, heart, brain, sinuses. A spinal tap. Eye and dental exams. Neurocognitive and psychological evaluations. And repeated analysis of blood counts and urine, measuring some well-known components such as sodium and potassium, and other recondite metrics like the BUN-to-creatinine ratio and the anion gap. It is breathtaking simply to behold the volume of data one can harvest from the human body, the quantity of things that can be measured, and the precision with which those measurements are taken. And yet so much remains unknown. With every cubic centimeter of blood extracted from our child, the team was pushing forward into that darkness, both for his sake and for every patient's to come.

The time required for the pre-transplant workup—and to solve the lingering lung problem—gave us the opportunity to recover from the chaos of the move to Durham, adjust to the new environment, and gird ourselves for what was to come. Felicia quickly determined she preferred North Carolina to New York, I maintained enough of my Program to stay on track, and Lydia's teachers quickly declared her a "bloom where planted" child.

Thankfully, Sebastian adapted without a hiccup. On days when he didn't need to fast for one of the more involved procedures, he was reliably tranquil and positive. His PICC line was an inconvenience and the steroids made him red and puffy, but he managed everything with his typical élan. As a matter of daily routine, the hospital took the place of his preschool—it was the building filled with friendly grown-ups and familiar kids where he went every day from 9 a.m. to 2 p.m. There were games, activities, and even tests, albeit of a radically different nature and frequency.

It helped that we were not alone. As previously mentioned, the patient population is a sizable constituency in the neighborhoods near the hospital, providing a built-in sense of belonging and solidarity. Over the course of our visits we were getting acquainted with other transplant kids. They seemed to be handling things just as smoothly as Sebastian. It's often said the process is harder on the parents than on the patients—the dignity and grace with which the children at Duke were facing their treatment would have impressed Nelson Mandela.

In the upstairs unit of our town house at Alden Place, the family of a fourteen-year-old girl named Khaleda was going through hell. Khaleda was struggling to make it after an agonizing effort to cure yet another crazy and cruel disease I'd never heard of: beta-thalassemia major, a hemoglobin disorder that leads to severe anemia, growth disorders, and organ failure. Born in Afghanistan, Khaleda was diagnosed at two and required regular blood transfusions to survive. In 2009, she'd been adopted by a North Carolina couple named Amanda and Mike Assell. They'd recently suffered a miscarriage and, with complete knowledge of Khaleda's condition and outlook, they opened their hearts and their home to her, committing their lives to getting her the treatment she could never have gotten in her war-torn homeland. The odds for a successful transplant were mediocre at best, but it was Khaleda's best hope for making it to adulthood. Her parents signed each page of their own patient treatment plan, counting on the Duke team to work its wonders.

Things had not gone well. A first transplant failed, then a second. Khaleda spent more than four months on the Unit, weeks of them in intensive care after she developed a bacterial lung infection in an immunosuppressed state. Now, if only her old immune system could recover enough, she could return to her old normal and try to keep living with her disease. Khaleda handled all these horrible setbacks without complaint or blame. In the meantime, her parents, racked with exhaustion and second-guessing, sustained themselves with their deep, unabashed Christianity.

Overt display of faith was common, if not prevalent, in Durham, where the standard opposition between the scientific and the spiritual is commonly regarded as a false dichotomy. I was not surprised to hear many parents invoking the Lord's name with regularity in conversation and social media. The devotion of the staff, however, was a distinct difference from our experience in New York. The Duke nurses are fluent in the language of modern medicine; yet many (not all, but many) are also deeply religious—meaning Christian—and uninhibited about discussing their faith if the invitation presents itself. One, known as Crazy Marie, even followed Felicia into the ladies' room just to tell her God loves her. I don't know how that plays with the Saudis and Orthodox Jews who've come for transplant, but for Felicia, it was an unqualified plus.

Indeed, part of Felicia's adaptation to North Carolina was putting her faith into overdrive. Unfettered by the secular pressures of the yupper-class Northeast, she went all in. She joined a local church group. Soon every random, warmhearted stranger became an angel, every piece of good medical news a miracle. Soon every horizontal surface in our apartment was decorated with books on spirituality. Christian talk radio filled the living room round the clock. One of the large closets became her prayer "war room," its walls covered with Post-it notes with Scripture quotes and images to help guide her intercessions.

"I prayed for healing, I prayed to stay calm," Felicia said. She needed to believe in a higher power because she feared the lower powers at her disposal were not enough for the task at hand. "Belief in the divine makes it possible to imagine achievement and potential beyond your limitations and the restraints of your circumstances," she said. God also helped her with acceptance. "So much of our unhappiness is re-lated to trying to control things out of our dominion. Through prayer and meditation, I could distinguish between what was in my control and what was not."

It was clear to me that my wife needed to go heavy on the Lord to sus-tain herself through this process, and, as we were all depending on her strength, I wasn't going to object. (I'd also been personally re-sponsible for some of her anguish, so I was in no position to object to her remedy.) If Felicia broke down, there was no plan B. I had my pro-gram, she had hers. Whatever works.

My issue with evangelical Christianity wasn't the Christianity, it was the evangelizing—Felicia, truly believing our lives and our mar-riage would be much improved if we were spiritually aligned, repeat-edly tried to bring me along. She'd seize control of the car stereo and slide in religious CDs. She'd devote our date nights to watching Ken-drick Brothers movies. And she openly critiqued my choices in books, music, or TV if she thought they were polluting my mind. It was be-coming a problem.

"It saddens me that we can't share this journey of faith together. Why don't you try it? At the very least, you may be more fun to be around."

"You want me to believe in God to make you happy?"

"No, to make *you* happy. It seems that few things do."

"I'm not going to apologize for taking things seriously," I said. "Somebody has to take an analytical approach and prepare for whatever could go wrong. Counting on 'miracles' doesn't work for me."

"But we will *always* have terrible what-ifs in life, especially as Sebastian's parents. You'd have a more convincing argument if you at least seemed happy."

"Honestly, I'd be more open to your faith if you didn't lay it on so thick. Your hard sell turns me off to God like Greenpeace turns me off to environmental activism."

And so on. In the past, living in a house with this degree of Bible-thumping would eventually have led to a Category 5 rage episode. Whatever the proposed benefits of faith Felicia was touting, I objected morally to ascribing every good turn of events to divine intervention. For one thing, it belittled the efforts of our doctors and the sacrifices of previous patients. Secondly, the flip side of the logic was just cruel. If Khaleda didn't make it, would that mean God was punishing her family? If Sebastian didn't make it, would my lack of faith be to blame?

Fortunately, I'd acquired a skill that comes naturally to some people, but that took me years on my Program to develop: shutting up and walking away. On the drive down to North Carolina I'd sworn to keep our marital issues in check. I wasn't going to allow myself to do anything to stress out Sebastian, and my self-control in the aftermath of our recent home invasion was proof I could keep cool. In this situation, domestic harmony had to take precedence over winning a theological debate. "The only kind of man that argues with his wife is one who likes to be wrong," Hunter Glass advised. So when these conversations approached the border between discussion and argument, I just smiled, nodded, and found some excuse to do something else. It would have been easier to chew glass.

That ongoing exercise in equanimity was paired with an equally novel exercise in humility. The financial strains of the situation—though I emphatically acknowledge they were a trifle compared to what other families faced—were sufficiently egregious for us to sign up with COTA, the Children's Organ Transplant Association, which helps raise and distribute tax-deductible donations for families like ours. The group gets much less publicity than the GoFundMe campaigns some families launch, but it screens all clients and their expenses, so donors know their cash isn't subsidizing Lucky Strikes, lotto tickets, and hotel pay-per-view porn. The humbling part was telling the world—friends, colleagues, my old meditation sangha, the world of Facebook—that we weren't just PWASK, we were PWASK who needed money.

As we steeled ourselves for transplant, I had to break away and head to Philadelphia. In the wake of her cancer diagnosis, my mother was having part of her colon and small intestine removed. By now I was a pro at guiding a loved one through surgery and had become numb to many of the shocks that rattle the rookies. The poignancy of seeing my mom prepped for the table, her aging body sheathed in the flimsy robe, was leavened by the knowledge that at least this was natural—the old get ill, the young care for them. This was what a forty-five-year-old man was supposed to be doing—navigating Hospitalworld for his seventy-two-year-old mother, not his young son. She made it through without incident and encouraged me to head back to Durham days later, but I still felt like a turd for leaving her.

A few weeks later we celebrated Sebastian's birthday with a trip to the Outer Banks. Usually patients aren't supposed to travel more than a half hour's drive from the hospital, and with steroids suppressing his immune system Sebastian was at greater risk for infection; still, Prasad granted a special dispensation, with a stern admonition to call the 24-hour hotline if anything went wrong. Our hotel on Ocracoke Island was a five-hour drive and a ferry ride away—not the ideal place to have a rare-disease complication pre-transplant—but this would be our last family vacation for a long while, perhaps forever. It was worth the push.

Sebastian was four. We'd gotten him this far. As he ran along the beaches of Ocracoke, chasing plovers and killdeer, we were a happy, united family. As we celebrated the precious moment together, we finally felt ready. Unafraid.

When we returned to the Alden Place apartments our building was quieter than usual. "Come look at this," Felicia said later that night as she checked Facebook on her laptop, her hands over her mouth.

Khaleda had died on Mother's Day. Her mother posted a heartbreaking tribute on the family blog, detailing Khaleda's love of weddings, her dreams, and her suffering. The family found a way to find joy in her memory and make sense of her loss through their understanding of God's will, but it was certainly not the outcome they'd envisioned. It was a shock for all of us.

I would later learn that the nurses on the Unit observe special rituals when children are discharged. They line the hallways, cheer, and throw confetti as the patient makes his/her way toward the exit door. These are ecstatic, victorious moments. But not every kid leaves that way—some never make it out alive. When that happens, the nurses line the halls and pay their respects as the patient is wheeled out, draping the gurney in a special quilt decorated by the staff.

Khaleda was one of those kids. Her parents had always known her odds were long, and her disease had no relation to Sebastian's, but the glow of his birthday festivities soon dimmed under this somber reality.

A creeping sense of urgency built up over the following weeks. The longer we had to wait to be admitted, the more time there was for some other issue to pop up. It was now two full months since we'd first arrived in Durham, plenty of time to shift gears from Where the Hell Are We? to Bring It On! We'd picked our favorite restaurants, transitioned from Stop & Shop to Harris Teeter, and adjusted to the horizontality of life in a landscape without skyscrapers. Everything was in place—we just needed medical clearance for takeoff. A great Geto Boys lyric said it all: "If it's goin' down, then let's get this shit over with!"

Sebastian was scheduled for his next CT scan on May 23 to see if the nodules had cleared. This was the make-or-break test that would determine if Prasad's decision to switch to steroids was correct. I was growing concerned about the cumulative effect of all the radiography bombarding my son's thorax—kids are more sensitive to radiation than adults and a *New York Times* article I'd read characterized frequent X-rays as a good recipe for cancer. "The long-term risks are negligible," Prasad assured me. "In any case, there is no choice—we need to know the lungs are clear before we admit for transplant."

There is no drier language than the prose of medical test results. In this case, to us, the arid sentences of the radiology report were as soaring as Keats couplets: "No effusion or pneumothorax. Central airways are patent. Resolved right upper lobe atelectasis. Scattered bilateral pulmonary nodules, many which have decreased in size or resolved compared to prior." That is all ye know on earth, and all ye need to know.

The case of the mystery Q-tips was solved, Prasad's hunch vindicated, the denouement worthy of Arthur Conan Doyle as we Watsons stood agog at the great man's powers of deductive reasoning.

That medical masterstroke was still fresh in our minds when, one week later, Dr. Prasad passed us the pen to sign each page of the treatment plan. I looked into his chocolate eyes and saw the self-assurance of a fighter pilot. Khaleda had died on his unit days earlier, and now, without flinching, he was ready for whatever came next. Felicia could have her deity; I had mine.

The document in front of us was more than a waiver or a schedule. It was the synthesis of all the fastidious probes that had consumed the past months, the genetic matching of Sebastian's HLA typing with the donor units in the cord blood bank, and microliter-precise calculations of the proper dosages for the countless medicines to come. The plan represented the cracking of a code, the true solution to a puzzle that had bedeviled us since Sebastian's first fever back in 2012. "The pre-transplant planning is arguably more vital to success than the transplant itself," said Prasad. "We've looked for any active or hidden infections, we've assessed the patient's ability to tolerate chemo, and we've arrived at the best way to minimize risks while maximizing the odds the transplant will take." There were still dozens of things that could go wrong—as we could plainly see—but the Duke team had anticipated almost everything and was equipped with a vast arsenal of effective countermeasures.

"If I may quote Gary Gilmore," I said after signing the final page, "let's do it."

On the eve of our admission, Sebastian and Felicia were running through grass near one of the playgrounds at Alden Place. Their variation of tag required her to chase him, then swoop in to pick him up and swing him around while tickling his tummy. Every time she did, the air rippled with his peals of laughter as he savored the fun and safety of his mother's arms, throwing his newsboy-capped head back with abandon. He'd been told repeatedly what was about to happen, but in the moment, he either didn't care or didn't comprehend. As the sun set, his final minutes of ignorant bliss expired.

He arrived at the hospital at 7 a.m. on June 3, packed as one might for a camping trip. The parent handbook we'd scoured listed everything we should bring, stressing that the Unit's claustrophobic quarters made it imperative to pack light. One week's worth of clothes, washed twice and carried in clean plastic bags; basic toiletries; slippers; favorite toys, books, and pillow. Personal decorations were encouraged; live plants and balloons strictly forbidden.

The experience was reminiscent of a hotel check-in, except at this five-star property, all guests require surgery before gaining access to their rooms. This procedure was not to remedy any illness or injury but to install new equipment inside Sebastian's body to facilitate the transplant process. He'd be spending the coming months as a semi-cybernetic organism, a four-year-old fusion of biology and technology.

The most important piece of gear was the central line, a catheter inserted into a large vein in the chest leading directly to the heart. It functions as the primary access route into and out of the patient's body, enabling the team to administer chemotherapy, medicine, nutritional fluids, blood products, and infuse the donor cells. It also makes it possible to take the countless blood draws required to monitor the progress or regress of the entire process. "You can't do transplant without a central line, given the amount of medications involved," explained Prasad. "Not having a secure channel into the bloodstream would make it impossible; and with all the blood tests we have to do, we'd run out of veins in two days. It's actually one of the unsung heroes of transplantation."

The central line was the major-league version of the PICC line it now replaced—same function, but designed for a more heavy-duty workload. Its main tube forked out into three separate tributary lines called lumens, each with its own IV port. For a period of indeterminate length, Sebastian would live with this tube dangling out of his chest, and—crucially—it needed to be cared for meticulously to prevent tangling, breakage, or contamination, despite anticipated contact with vomit, blood, and/or human waste.

The second piece of new plumbing was a nasogastric (NG) tube, run up through the nose and down into the esophagus. Its purpose: to deliver adequate nutrition after the chemo obliterated the lining of our child's digestive tract and he could no longer swallow food.

To prepare him for all this, one of the child life specialists had met with Sebastian weeks earlier. She'd shown him a central line, encouraged him to play with it, and let him insert a feeding tube into a doll's nose.

Now it was showtime.

Pediatric surgery was on the third floor of the children's hospital. Felicia and Sebastian arrived early for prep. I followed shortly with Lydia after attending her second-grade graduation. We sat in our accustomed posture in the waiting room, eyes transfixed on monitors on which each patient's status was displayed and updated like departing flights. Sebastian's progressed agonizingly from "prep" to "anesthesia" to "operating." I left the room and strolled over to the walkway overlooking the open atrium of the Children's Hospital—its glazed, multistoried courtyard space almost tricked me into thinking we were on a cruise ship, polluting the Caribbean as we steamed from Cozumel to Belize City, a swarm of overfed Americans attacking the buffet.

Felicia appeared and summoned me back to the waiting room. The status field on the monitor had advanced to "recovery." A bearded surgeon, who might have been the World's Most Interesting Man from the Dos Equis ad campaign, explained that everything had gone smoothly; we could head to Sebastian's bedside in the recovery room to await his revival.

We'd been through this five times by my count, enough for portions of the process to feel routine. The "novelty" this time was that the child we saw knocked out in the bed, the kid who'd been running and laughing in a playground the day before, now had these two new tubes extending like rubber tendrils out of his chest and nose. Our Pinocchio now had strings. This is what we'd signed up for.

Just wake up . . . just wake up. . . . I silently incanted my traditional recovery room mantra for a twenty-minute eternity until he came to, crying in discomfort from the intrusion of the NG tube. The internal portion of the tube was lodged permanently in the back of his throat like a partially swallowed fettuccine noodle. Its external portion was taped to the side of his face. Our efforts to prepare him mentally notwithstanding, he was scared and miserable.

We were told that in a day or two his throat would feel fine. In the meantime, we headed to the Unit. Room 5214 had been prepared for us; the nurses were ready to receive.

There are sixteen patient rooms on the L-shaped unit. The patient census typically hovers between five and fourteen; when we rolled in it stood at about ten. The door to each patient's room is decorated with the occupant's name spelled out in construction-paper letters, various pictures and drawings, and—for those whose donor cells have engrafted—a customized poster marking the date and blood counts on the all-important day.

Felicia had spent weeks here back in March but many of the details were still fresh for me. Immediately I noticed the almost comic diversity of the families. To mention a few whose names I've changed, there was Clara, whose parents were lab researchers from Boston; LeVonna, the infant daughter of a single black mother from Virginia; Ameena, a hijabbed teenage girl from the United Arab Emirates; Tucker, a white kid from one of the RC Cola zones below the Mason-Dixon. We were the cast of a four-quadrant disaster flick.

To understand the culture of the Unit, think of a submarine, a prison, or the International Space Station. Any place where people are forced to live together in confinement under precarious circumstances. Most of life takes place in the tiny patient rooms, but patients' families can mingle in the common areas. There's a Connection Room with toys and games for the kids cleared to be in public; a parent space for caregiver rest and relaxation; and a kitchen area equipped with a fridge, microwave, stove, and sink. Each family can store and prepare (individually labeled) groceries there, with the iron rule that all dishes must be scrubbed and placed in the high-powered washer. There was a small laundry room, decorated with a detailed sign describing a rigorous decontamination process to be used on the washers and dryers before and after use. Each patient room had its own bathroom, absolutely off-limits for anyone but the patient. Caregivers used a shared commode and shower, which had to undergo disinfection before and after each use. The parents knew the dangers and respected them—many grew adept at raising the toilet seat and flushing with their feet. If we could have wiped with our feet, we would have.

Katie Burke, another nurse on Sebastian's team, was on duty when we moved into room 5214, plastic bags of clothes and toys in tow. Like a perky real estate agent showing a Manhattan studio, she gave the full tour in twenty seconds.

Then she moved on to the daily routine that would now define our waking and sleeping lives. It involved a daily bath, a morning weigh-in, taking of vital signs every four hours, application of cardiac leads and a pulse oximeter while sleeping, central line care, walks and exercise on the Unit, playtime, naps, and if needed, physical and speech therapy.

"And over heeeere," Katie continued, turning to the counter sink above a mini-fridge by the door, "we have the setup for the oral hygiene procedure." Four times a day, she explained, the caregiver had to execute a special mouth care routine to prevent chemo-related sores. On the sink she placed bottles of sodium bicarbonate, Peridex antibacterial solution, and chlorhexidine mouth rinse. "After every meal and before bedtime," she said, hoisting a stick with a green sponge brush on one end called a Toothette, "you need to soak one of these in each of the solutions and rub them over his teeth and gums." One nightly rinse with fluoride was also mandatory.

"Why can't we use his normal toothbrush?" I asked.

"The chemo degrades the tissues in the mouth. Scrubbing with a toothbrush would rupture the tissue and cause bleeding. He won't have any platelets for a while, so the bleeding wouldn't stop." She knew enough of these horrors to describe them offhandedly, but her point was made.

These routines were all sideshows to the main event—the administration of intravenous medications. Most of these would be pumped straight into Sebastian's heart through the central line in precise dosages. Each medication would be delivered, usually over the course of several hours, through its own infusion pump. The pumps, in turn, attached in branches to a single metal pole. The pole itself, towering over the bed, loomed as Sebastian's protector, his jailer, his cross. It would not leave his side for two months.

The transplantation process, I realized, would be a total team effort. This was not a discrete event like a surgery, with preoperative, interoperative, and post-operative phases handled by separate staffs. A transplant is a round-the-clock operation lasting months, requiring a rotating crew of doctors, nurses, aides, and administrators, constantly monitoring dozens of different body functions, cell counts, and side effects. The astronaut comparison that applied during the pre-transplant testing was equally apt on the Unit, the central nurses' station serving as NASA mission control from which the journey of each patient would be tracked and adjusted on a day-to-day, hour-to-hour, sometimes minute-to-minute basis.

Felicia and I were a big part of that team. During previous hospital stays our sole purpose was to comfort and advocate for our son. Here on 5200, life would revolve around this demanding cycle of daily tasks, a to-do list that would not end. There would always be the next thing. This was a job.

Before the first day was out, there were more papers to sign—consent forms for three separate research studies. As we learned at NIH, each transplant patient is priceless. Sebastian's blood, his urine, even his poop were as precious as rare earth metals. We signed on without blinking—given all we were taking from the medical system, the least we could give back was some data.

Felicia was doing her best to address the helpless, questioning look in Sebastian's eyes by reminding him he was beginning a process of transformation. She'd taped her transplant cartoon panels to the wall and talked Sebastian through them. "Seeds become trees and caterpillars become butterflies," she explained in her airy soprano, "and little boys who need to take medicine turn into little boys who don't. But they all have to do scary stuff to change."

She'd had a long day. I volunteered to spend the first few nights on the Unit. Sebastian's throat was still sore from the surgery and he refused to eat. Before I performed the mouth care routine for the first time—which he detested—I convinced him to drink enough lemon-lime Gatorade that he had to pee. Like every other bodily function, his urine output had to be monitored, so I asked him to stand up in bed, unsheathe what we called "Samuel Johnson," and let fly into a plastic jug. Then I tucked him in and stroked his head as he fell asleep.

Tomorrow, with our signed consent, the doctors would start flooding his little body with toxic chemotherapy drugs. This was his last night as a caterpillar.

Chapter 11

Conditioning

....

Hospitalworld warps time, and it marks time differently too. Our first day on the Unit wasn't counted as Day 1, it was Day -13. This was all laid out on our road map, a custom calendar in spreadsheet form charting the medications and procedures to be administered each day in accordance with the treatment plan. Those thirteen negative-numbered days ticked off a two-week countdown to Day 0, Transplant Day—colloquially known as the patient's Rebirthday. During that time, Prasad and the team would put Sebastian through his chemotherapy regimen. How his little body handled that sustained assault would determine both the quality and quantity of the rest of his life.

There are more than one hundred approved chemotherapy drugs in use today, primarily for the treatment of cancer. Which ones a patient receives depends on the type, stage, and location of the cancer. Modern advances have made it possible to boost the chances of effective treatment while minimizing the odds of serious side effects, but the fundamental mechanism of chemotherapy hasn't changed from the blunt, brutal approach it's always been.

Here's how it works. Chemo kills cells that grow and divide rapidly. Cancer cells, notoriously, grow quickly and out of control, so they are particularly vulnerable to chemo. But fast-growing *healthy* cells get caught up in the culling too—these include those of the skin, the hair, the intestines . . . and white blood cells. That's why immune deficiency patients frequently go through chemo for transplant—they don't have cancer, but the chemo is a reliable way to eliminate the existing immune system.

Unfortunately, CGD patients typically require the most aggressive form of chemotherapy "conditioning," what's called "ablative" treatment. "The CGD kids have a very high incidence of graft failure. Even when using donor cells from perfectly matched siblings, we see a much higher rate of rejection," explained Dr. Kurtzberg. "We think it's because the rest of the immune system is compensating for the malfunctioning neutrophils. So it's harder to knock it out. We need to give them more medicine."

Over the years Duke has developed its own CGD-specific protocol. Thankfully it avoids the need for the harshest tool in the shed—total body irradiation—that carries a significant long-term risk of brain tumors, thyroid suppression, and effects on cognition. Instead, Sebastian's conditioning would start with three days of a drug called fludarabine, then four on the heavy-hitter busulfan, and four more on a third called Cytoxan. We'd soon become intimately acquainted with the unique profile of each.

On the morning of Day -12, nurse Liz Vaughn and one of the attending doctors entered the room with the first dose of fludarabine. Before the drug is administered, two doctors must separately review and sign off on the order and the dosage—the optimal dosage window is narrow, the consequences of miscalculation can be fatal. After dotting every *i* and crossing every *t*, the nurses hung the solution on Sebastian's pole and proceeded to pump poison into our child's chest. A heavy conditioning regimen is typically agonizing. "When he starts complaining of pain, we can manage that a bunch of different ways," Liz said, "everything from acetaminophen to a fentanyl drip."

Accustomed to the dramatic pacing of Shakespearean poisonings, I figured the barfing and moaning would ramp up within minutes. But no—fludarabine doesn't kill existing cells immediately. It simply inhibits mitosis, the mechanism by which their DNA replicates. Eventually, if the cells can't divide, they die. The patient typically feels nothing for days, until the other chemo drugs pile on.

The biggest immediate concern was how Sebastian's liver would process the medicine. Chemo is known to cause a rare and deadly condition called veno-occlusive disease (VOD) in which the veins in the liver get blocked. This is one of the most common, and lethal, complications from transplant. Anticipating that possibility, the road map called for a daily infusion of Actigall, a drug typically used to dissolve gallstones, which had become the go-to prophylaxis for VOD at Duke. The nurses hung another infusion pump on the pole next to the fludarabine and began another drip. He'd be on the Actigall every day until, *inshallah*, the last traces of chemo cleared his body a month later.

The foundational strategy of the entire process was now coming to light—determine the best drugs and dosages needed for transplant; anticipate their side effects and administer *another* layer of drugs to prevent or counteract them; anticipate the side effects of *those* drugs and be prepared to administer yet *another* set of drugs as further countermeasures, ad infinitum. Throughout the process, the team at mission control had to monitor blood count and chemistry, organ functions and vital signs, constantly on guard for warning signs. If action was required, the full toolbox of modern medicine was at the doctors' disposal.

One of the most important cautionary measures was the simplest—keep the body's systems up and running with regular intake of food and fluids. When the metabolism is humming along, it's easier to process out all those toxic chemicals and compounds. This is where parents can do more than watch and worry. By encouraging Sebastian to eat and drink regularly we were actively helping his body purge what are essentially poisons. At some point down the line he'd only be able to get nutrition through his NG tube, but as long as he could still chew and swallow normally, we were happy to cater to him. It felt good to be useful.

"Here's the shopping list," Felicia said as she went on duty later on Day -12. "Please make sure you get everything on it, and nothing else."

"Okay, so: Cheetos, Snickers, Oreos, Oscar Mayer salami, hot dogs, Kraft Mac and Cheese, Cool Ranch Doritos, Sprite. Sounds about right. I'm on it."

We were still getting our heads around the special diet mandated for transplant patients, which turned out to be another bizarre, through-the-looking-glass inversion of life on 5200. This neutropenic diet is built around two iron-clad mandates: consume calories by any means necessary and avoid food-borne illness at all costs—you really don't want to wrestle with an *E. coli* or salmonella infection without an immune system. Perversely, this meant many of the foods we normally think of as healthy were suddenly forbidden. Fresh fruit, vegetables, nuts, fresh deli meats and cheeses, herbs, spices including pepper, even some kinds of ice: all banned. Conversely, processed, preservative-laden, precooked crap we'd been avoiding assiduously for the past four years was now on the approved list. Chips, candy, mass-produced cookies, bottled soda, frozen pizza, Pop-Tarts, processed lunch meat, ketchup—bring it on. *Sayonara*, Whole Foods; *konnichiwa*, 7-Eleven. "There's a bit of controversy about the diet," one of the doctors told me later. "It's really based on common sense more than science."

Sebastian, his face now frequently speckled with Cheetos dust, was not about to question the protocol. The cuisine was a little kid's fantasy. Between that and an unlimited access to the TV and a stack of Thomas the Tank Engine DVDs, he was making himself at home. The discomfort in his throat from the NG tube had dissipated and the awkwardness of the central line was mitigated by a custom vest designed and sewn by a nurse named Marybeth Tetlow specifically for pediatric transplant patients to keep their tubes untangled and clean. (It's now patented and will soon be available commercially as the Line Snuggler. Next stop, *Shark Tank*.)

In that first week of chemo Sebastian was able to go "off the pole" for a good chunk of the day. The first medicines only dripped for a few hours, and some could be infused concurrently, so the schedule allowed some welcome breaks. Sebastian considered the pole both a physical hindrance and a public embarrassment, and so he relished these brief liberations. After the nurses disconnected his central line from the pole, he'd hop out of bed, put on a mask, and (after we wiped it down) hop on his beloved tricycle or into a red wagon for a ride.

His imprisonment had yet to sink in. "Mom," he asked Felicia, "when can we go outside?"

"We have to wait until we fix your blood, so that you can be healthy without taking medicine," she explained.

"But, Mommy, I *am* healthy!" he insisted. To prove it, he pedaled the trike as fast as he could past the doctors at the nurses' station to demonstrate his fitness and stamina.

That began to change shortly after Day -9, when Sebastian cycled off fludarabine and started his regimen of busulfan. The name itself sounds diabolical, and indeed the drug is classified as an alkylating agent—the family of compounds that includes mustard gas. This class of drug is ruthlessly effective at killing cells in their resting phase. Its signature side effect is seizures. To counteract that possibility, the road map called for the addition of an antiseizure medication called Keppra. Whether he was starting to feel the force of all the medications (Keppra changes electrical activity in the brain) or just adapting psychologically to the rhythms of life on the Unit, the net result on Sebastian was an overall dialing down of kinetic energy. He wasn't lethargic, just mellow, his mind's Pandora radio switched from Devo to Bread.

Outside his room, the other gears of the transplant process were engaging. Days before we'd been admitted, over at the Carolinas Cord Blood Bank, Dr. Kurtzberg had ordered the final round of testing and prep for our donor unit, the one with the beautiful five out of six HLA match. From the womb of a white, three-foot-high cylindrical robotic freezer, the unit emerged after years frozen in liquid nitrogen. Encased in a rectangular plastic wrapping, it could have been a vampire's frozen dinner. Stripped of all identifying information save a bar code, the packaging contained the main body of the sample plus three segments of cord blood stored separately for a final round of analysis prior to transplant. One of those segments had been detached and was now being assayed to confirm the potency of the unit. We were entering the final countdown.

My new workspace was ideally designed to absorb the impact of bad news—a bomb shelter for the mind. Management at the local affiliate had kindly agreed to let me work out of an unoccupied office up on the engineering floor, across from a large operations room crammed with servers, routers, and satellite dish replacement parts. With those indifferent machines as neighbors I was fortuitously segregated from the main newsroom—better not to be burrowed in an ant farm of cubicles and curious newsfolk when I felt the urge to weep or punch a wall.

The room was unwindowed, the walls bare. Old manuals and engineering schematics lined a metal bookcase. Since my arrival, papers and Post-its had spread like moss over the desk and credenza. I was in my natural corporate habitat. The only annoyance was that the mission-critical equipment across the hall required uncompromising climate control. With the air-conditioning on overdrive it felt like Oslo in October; outside, the summer sun had turned downtown Durham into a tandoor.

I was screening file footage when the office phone rang, to my instant consternation. I was expecting a call from Hunter Glass on the status of his investigation, but instead caller ID displayed the familiar 668 exchange of the Duke Hospital switchboard.

"Miguel, hi, I'm on with Dr. Kurtzberg and Dr. Prasad." It was Felicia, calm, serious, circumspect.

An unscheduled conference call with both doctors requiring the participation of both parents could mean only one thing: something was wrong.

"No emergency," said Kurtzberg, though by now I'd become a connoisseur of doctors' *brace yourself* voices, and this was assuredly hers. "It just that we've learned something about the donor units we need to share with you."

The news was a body blow. The potency assay measured a specific enzyme that correlates strongly with what they call CFUs, colony-forming units. The more CFUs, the better the chance of engraftment and a positive outcome.

The assay had been an abysmal failure. "The enzymes were close to zero, actually," said Kurtzberg. Something had probably gone wrong in the initial freezing process. "I'm sorry to tell you this but we believe it's unlikely these cells will engraft."

I took a moment and a cleansing breath to assess the damage of this bunker buster. *FUCK!* Sebastian had caught one and only one lucky break in our three-year donor search, this outstanding five out of six match. Suddenly, the golden ticket, which had given us the courage to embark on this ordeal, was a confirmed counterfeit. And now we were six days into chemo. There was no turning back.

Felicia stepped into the silence. "You're *sure* about that?"

Kurtzberg had parried reflexive denial before. "Yes. We repeated the test three times."

When I spoke, it was with the righteous rage of a swindled consumer calling out a bait-and-switch. "Why couldn't you have figured this out *before* we signed the consent forms and *before* you started napalming Sebastian's immune system with chemo?"

Kurtzberg tried to explain. They can't perform the potency assay until the unit is brought out of the freezer, which only happens just before conditioning begins. It takes several days to complete the test, so they never get results until chemo has already started. The overlap isn't usually a problem because it's rare that a good-looking donor unit like ours turns out to be a dud.

"Believe me, I wish there were some easier answer," added Kurtzberg meekly. "Then you wouldn't yell at me."

I composed myself and apologized. "Please forgive me. I just can't tell you how tired we are of surprises regarding our son's health."

"So we see two options," Prasad intervened, "which I can explain to you in better detail when I see you tomorrow morning on the Unit. The good news is we have some time to decide. Okaayyy?"

Fifteen minutes later I was en route to pick up Lydia from her Elysium of a summer day camp, while a half tab of Klonopin was en route to my stomach. In the rented Dodge Caravan, aftershocks from the phone call reverberated in my head and coalesced into a single, thundering thought: *It's not going to work, he's not going to make it.* Heeding the mindfulness training, I tried to focus on the breath coming in and out of my nostrils, but—apologies to Thich Nhat Hanh—it wasn't until Captain K crossed the blood-brain barrier and went to work that I felt any measure of relief.

By the time I pulled up at the camp parking lot I was ready to play Strong Daddy. Lydia, as usual, was a fountain of positivity as she strapped in. "Dad, today was *awe*-some! We got to swim in the river, we dug for bugs, and then after lunch we played wilderness tag."

"You sprayed with Off, right?" Captain K had vanquished the panic, not the lugubriousness.

"Mm-hmm."

"And you put on extra sunblock in the afternoon?"

"Yes, Dad."

It's not going to work, he's not going to make it.

"Dad, did you go to camp?"

"Eh . . . yes and no. I went to camps, but not like this. Music camp, physics camp. Basically, geek camp."

"I'd like to do that too."

"Sure, sweetie. But you know, it's fine if you don't. You don't have to be like me."

"What if I *want* to be like you?"

I took my eyes off the road and looked at her beautiful face. Soon enough she'd be a teenager hating my guts, but for the moment I was her idol, whether I deserved to be or not. *So, let's try to deserve it.*

We made it up to the 5200 and buzzed in. I was still getting used to the strict policy of *never* touching the door handles and pressing elevator buttons with knuckles. Someone had also told us to minimize contact with cash—another common disease vector. As Lydia and I slipped paper booties over our shoes, scrubbed our hands, and donned face masks I tried to prepare myself mentally for the jump from Healthyworld to Hospitalworld.

We'd done this dozens of times already, but entering the Unit still felt like Keanu Reeves disconnecting from the Matrix. The abrupt change in the physical environment was only part of it. In Healthyworld trivial things could put on airs of urgency—Did I need a haircut? Was Elizabeth Warren finally going to start stumping for Hillary? In

Hospitalworld the only things that mattered were Sebastian's vital signs and daily blood work. The contrast between the two worlds was amplified by the fact that one child was inhabiting each. In Healthyworld there lived a daughter about to celebrate her eighth birthday, practicing piano, hunting for frogs at camp. In Hospitalworld there lived a son trying to make it through each day of chemo without his internal organs turning to applesauce.

The HEPA filters in the patient rooms can get overloaded with too many visitors, so we weren't spending much time there together as a family. Like runners in an Olympic relay with two alternating baton bearers, Felicia and I had an immense sense of shared commitment to a common goal, but only fleeting moments of human contact. Some days we'd hang out together for an hour or two, but she didn't appreciate my company when I was stressing, so on days like today it was going to be a quick handoff.

As Lydia and I walked into the room Felicia was lying in the bed next to Sebastian, reading him a poignant, therapeutic children's book called *It Will Be Okay* by Lysa TerKeurst. It tells the story of two friends, Little Seed and Little Fox, who together deal with the trauma of the seed being planted, spending an extended period in the subterranean cold and dark, and finally emerging as a strong, striving plant. The fox stands over the soil the entire time, reassuring the frightened seed by repeating the book's title. *It Will Be Okay* was one of several ways Felicia was trying to explain what was happening. It seemed to work.

It was still a shock for me to see my beloved son with his twin tentacles—feeding tube up his nose, central line dangling out of his chest—and the IV pole, now laden with five different infusion pumps, looming over him like a scarecrow. There'd be no detaching from it now.

But none of it seemed to bother him today. As his eyes turned from the book pages to the doorway and he saw who was entering the room, he sat up in bed, shouted, "Yayyyy!" and began a game of Hungry Hungry Hippos with his sister. Everything Kurtzberg and Prasad had told us about the sustaining power of sibling companionship, which I'd previously pooh-poohed, suddenly made perfect sense. Lydia was Sebastian's best and only friend, the one person whose presence allowed him to be a kid, not just a patient. (Another mother from the Unit later told me that, after her daughter went into a troubling sleep for three straight days, Prasad called for an older sister to come into the room. The patient regained consciousness within hours.)

As the kids played, Felicia and I stepped outside.

"Promise me you'll stay positive tonight." This was my wife in coach mode. "Keep his spirits up. Don't let your anxiety scare him. He can smell it."

"Fair enough."

After the girls left I prepared Sebastian's favorite dinner—Kraft Mac & Cheese, salami slices, and Skittles—and rolled the meal under his chin on the adjustable plastic table next to the bed. To wash it all down I poured a cocktail we called Special Mix—Orangina and lemon-lime Gatorade—served reverentially in a Styrofoam cup clearly marked with his name. On 5200, sipping from someone else's straw can be a dreadful mistake.

He fed himself while watching a Thomas the Tank Engine video aptly titled *Tale of the Brave* and I took a moment to review the road map. It stretched out to Day 365. We were only on Day -6 and I shook my head as I contemplated the minefield immediately ahead. Tomorrow would be the last day of busulfan, with the scheduled rotation onto Cytoxan coming right after. Then there'd follow a mother-of-all-bombs immunosuppressant called ATG (antithymocyte globulin) that they pour on at the end. The nastiest side effects were still weeks away, but in addition to the current risk of liver failure and seizures, we'd soon have to contend with nausea, possible kidney failure, hives, and diarrhea.

Deal with what's in front of you.

I put away the road map as the door swung open. "Hey, guyyyys, how we doin'?" It was Katie the night shift nurse, as upbeat and on-task as a homeroom teacher on Monday morning. She tapped the hand sanitizer dispenser by the door and walked to the bed to check vital signs. The overhead monitor had been tranquil all day—heart rate hovering around 106 beats per minute and oxygen saturation steady at 99 percent. Nevertheless, every four hours the nurses had to check the other vitals: blood pressure and temperature. Especially temperature—fever meant infection, infection meant trouble.

"Hey, got something for ya." I squeezed into the bathroom and came out bearing a small plastic jug sloshing with the output of Sebastian's last pee. "Two hundred and fifty milliliters. We're quite proud." After a dozen infusions of busulfan, it was vital for his little kidneys to filter the toxins out of his blood and purge them from his system. (We'd later learn what happens when the chemo drugs linger.) The fact that he'd wizzed out more than a fourth of a 7-Eleven Big Gulp was a victory. Best of all—no blood.

"I peed in a juuuugg!" declared Sebastian. After nearly three months in North Carolina he'd adopted the elongated vowels of Dixie.

"Great job, buddy!" Kate leaned in for a high five. As she spoke she began the daily chore of replacing the caps on his central line ports, her dexterous fingers hovering over his chest like hummingbirds. "Just a heads-up—it's going to be kind of a busy night in here 'cause we got a bunch of drips cycling on and off. The mesna runs every four hours, in sync with the vitals. The last dose of busulfan starts around nine p.m. That should end around two in the morning, and you get a loading dose of Keppra with that. Blood draw is at midnight as usual."

I was curious why everything had to go through the IV—I'd looked up mesna and Keppra and knew they were also given orally. "It's because chemo can cause vomiting," she explained. "We can't have other med-icines in the stomach—if he throws them up he'd miss a dose." 'Nuff said.

It was lights-out at 9 p.m., and if there's one positive thing to say about fully ablative chemotherapy it's that the fatigue it induces helps kids go right to sleep at bedtime. With Sebastian down, I braced myself for another night of combat with the sleeping arrangements.

With proper bedding and positioning, falling asleep was manage-able. Staying asleep was another matter. Whenever there was a dis-ruption in the drip or one of the infusions completed, the pump would start beeping, requiring attention from the nurse. The constant cy-cling of the various IV meds made sleeping in the room like spending the night amid a fleet of Home Depot forklifts, and with every beeping came a visit from Katie, a hatchet of hallway light hitting my face as the door swung open. Supplementing those external disturbances, that afternoon's conversation with Prasad and Kurtzberg was still clanging between my ears, loudly enough to spring me upright at about 3:30 a.m., fumbling in the dark for another half tab of help from Captain K.

It's not going to work; he's not going to make it.

As I looked across to the other side of Sebastian's bed I saw Katie there. She wasn't doing anything—no vitals, no meds—just standing over him in the dark like a guardian angel, her right hand on her heart, as if the vital signs monitor had been playing Whitney Houston's ren-dition of the national anthem. "He's so beautiful when he sleeps," she said as she turned her gaze to me, eyes moist with tears. "And you're so lucky. You get to be his daddy."

After three more hours of fitful slumber I awoke, looking like I'd spent the night under a bridge. Sebastian was still asleep at 7 a.m. and I was playing chess on my iPhone in a ratty T-shirt, gym shorts, and flip-flops when Dr. Prasad came in, immaculately groomed and parting the seas with his hyperachiever smile. It was early for him—daily rounds began after the morning staff meeting. He was here to see me, not the patient.

"Miguel, might we step outside and chat about the issue with the donor units? I have some paperwork I'd like to show you."

We moved out to the small nurses' station in the hall and settled into a pair of swivel chairs. On the far wall hung a "Today I Feel . . ." poster composed of dozens of cartoon children's faces, each representing a different emotion. Today I felt . . . exasperated.

"So as we discussed yesterday," Prasad began, "the potency assay on the primary unit came back low and we now believe it's unlikely these cells will engraft. That raises the question of the backup unit."

With every transplant, Duke requires two compatible units—a primary and the backup. We'd focused solely on the primary, that thrilling five out of six match. The backup had aced the potency assay, but it was a bottom-of-the-barrel four out of six. In my mind the difference was Jimmy Choo and Payless.

Or perhaps not. Prasad pulled out a sheet of paper with data on both units. "As you can see," he explained, "the primary—the five out of six match—is fully matched with Sebastian's type at the A-level locus, which is why it would normally be considered a better match than the backup unit. But I also want to show you this"—moving his finger over to the far-right column of the data table, where the raw size of the unit, the number of viable cells, was listed. "The cell dose per kilo on the backup unit is quite high—one hundred seven per kilogram of Sebastian's weight. Given that high dose, and the high potency of this backup unit, we're still confident of Sebastian's chances of success with the backup unit. Okaaay?" This was his thing—administering heavy doses of the word "okay" as an antidote to awkwardness.

"You'd said on the phone yesterday there were different options to consider."

"Yes. Now, the potency assay of the *primary* unit, as we said, was not good. We think if we were to go that route there would only be about a twenty percent chance of engraftment."

"It sounds like the backup unit is the only real choice."

"Not exactly. We often do *double* transplants, using *both* the primary *and* backup units on the same patient. Usually it's when we're transplanting larger teenagers, who obviously weigh more, and we *need* both units to achieve an adequate cell dose. We could try that with Sebastian and hope that twenty percent chance of the primary unit cells engrafting comes through. If not, the cells from the backup unit would be in there too. So overall we'd be increasing the odds of engraftment."

"What's the downside?"

"Okay, so the potential downside is that with a double transplant we'd be giving him such a large dose of donor cells from the combined units that he'd be getting many he doesn't need. That increases the likelihood of other problems. In particular it raises the probability of graft-versus-host disease."

"So what's *your* inclination?"

"I'm leaning toward trying the double. We started the process with that five out of six match in mind and tailored the conditioning regimen based on that, so I think we should try to make it work. That's *my* opinion."

"What's *Dr. Kurtzberg's* opinion?"

"Dr. Kurtzberg . . . feels we should play it safe and go with the backup unit alone."

It really came down to which bad outcome we most wanted to avoid—a failed engraftment or a severe case of GvHD. "Please don't tell me you're just going to throw this decision in our laps," I begged, hemorrhaging worry.

"No, no," he assured me. "In situations like this we take the data to the Monday meeting with the entire team. We will discuss and reach a consensus about what's best for the patient. Then we will inform you of our recommendation, but the final decision will be yours."

We left it at that. As I crept back into the room, one of the IV pumps was beeping. Sebastian was still zonked out and oblivious. Morning light was gushing through the window. It was going to be a sunny summer day in Healthyworld. In Hospitalworld, just like every other day, there was no weather.

I pressed the call button and waited for Katie to come in—sometimes she arrived in seconds; if she was busy elsewhere, it was like waiting for Windows 98 to start up. As the beeping persisted like an unanswered phone I caught myself licking a discolored lump that had formed on the right interior surface of my lower lip. Apparently I'd been biting my lip with such force and frequency I'd ruptured a vein and created what's known as a mucocele. Now I'd developed a weird habit—some might call it a tic—of rubbing my tongue against the red-black nodule. If you observed me in action with a few days' stubble on my chin, you'd likely mistake me for a deranged homeless dude squeegeeing windshields at the mouth of the Lincoln Tunnel.

A second IV pump started beeping and my mind began bouncing off the walls.

It's not going to work; he's not going to make it.

That little chat with Prasad meant we were in uncharted and turbulent waters. Up to this point he and Kurtzberg had always spoken in perfect unison. Now, on the vital matter of the donor unit itself, the two wizards were of different minds. By definition, that meant one of them was wrong, and aside from flipping a coin I had no way to determine which.

A glance down at my child, still silent and only half awake, but now blinking his brown eyes, the lashes as long as Betty Boop's. A few strands of his hair had fallen onto the pillow.

Pan over to the plastic table. Felicia had left the book there faceup.
Say the words:

"It will be okay."

"It WILL be okay."

"Itwillbeokayitwillbeokayitwillbeokay. . . ."

Chapter 12

Happy Rebirthday

About the meeting itself, we know very little. Around 8 a.m. on Monday, June 14, the doctors assembled for their biweekly conference and discussed the competing options for Sebastian's transplant, given the dilemma of the impotent primary unit. If voices were raised or tables pounded, those details didn't leave the room, though one doctor told me it's not unusual for things to get contentious. "People are very passionate," the doctor said. "That's why these meetings happen behind closed doors."

The conclave reached its decision before lunch. I was half expecting to see white smoke billowing from the roof of the hospital. Kurtzberg's plan carried the day: a single-dose transplant using the potent but imperfect four out of six matched backup unit. Prasad's preference, doing a double with the beautiful but feeble five out of six unit mixed in, had been voted down.

The outcome was no surprise. Prasad ran the Unit, but Kurtzberg maintained supreme authority regarding the pairing of patients with donor cells. The matching technique is an art as well as a science, she explained. "We screen five to ten units for every patient, and we look at many different factors. Some are obvious—the cell dose, the match, the potency test, the quality of the bank where the units were stored.

But how much weight should each factor carry? Everybody has their own algorithm as to what to prioritize."

One doctor on the team told me later that Kurtzberg's call with Sebastian was gutsy, borderline swashbuckling. "It's a controversial decision—seventy-five percent of the transplant centers wouldn't have gone forward with that unit. Their prior experience with single-dose four out of six matches is not good and they wouldn't think they'd be serving the patient well. Most likely they'd refer the patient to us instead, which is why we get patients from all over."

Not knowing this at the time, I was simply relieved they'd settled on a plan, even if it was a gambit. Felicia had the Lord to help sustain her; I'd put all my faith in these doctors and their science. The schismatic rumblings between Prasad and Kurtzberg on this matter had cracked the foundation of that faith. The decision spackled those cracks over, and now, as a unified team, we could confront the next challenge. . . .

Which was a head-scratcher. The whole purpose of chemo conditioning is to wipe out the patient's white blood cells, but after ten straight days of regular, relentless doses, Sebastian's cell counts were still hovering in the normal range. Added to that, very little of his hair had fallen out. It didn't make sense. "I can promise you we *gave* him the chemo drugs," said a bemused Dr. Kristin Page, the attending physician that week, as she reviewed that day's labs. "We'll see what happens with the ATG."

She was referring to the last of the conditioning drugs, a peculiar medicine derived from horse or rabbit hormones that has proven breathtakingly effective at suppressing the human immune system. *How* it does this is still partially unknown—some of the suggested mechanisms of action are hypothetical—but *what* it does is clear. ATG is the equivalent of the Air Force's legendary "Daisy Cutter"—a bomb so strong it can single-handedly flatten a section of forest into a helicopter landing zone.

Sure enough, by Day -2, ATG and the chemo had completed the extermination campaign. The floor dropped out of Sebastian's white blood count. That day's labs showed the counts for neutrophils, lymphocytes, monocytes, and all the other cells plummeting toward John Blutarsky's grade point average: 0.0.

Sebastian was now, for the first time, officially in the boy-in-the-bubble state, his body utterly defenseless against infection of any kind, just as it was being taxed as never before. A total of six medicines were pumping into his heart throughout the day, including one to prevent kidney bleeding; and, as predicted, their cumulative impact was taking a toll on his digestive system.

The diarrhea began—first as a trickle, soon as a mud volcano. We'd had such a tempestuous history with this kid's butt and feces already—I briefly considered titling this book *Blood, Shit, and Tears*—I instantly imagined another perirectal abscess blossoming now, at the worst possible moment. I didn't panic, but I implored the nurses for a solution. The first thing they suggested, as a matter of basic hygiene, was to switch him from underwear to diapers immediately.

I once read a book about the ethnic conflicts in Dagestan. Its author argued that subjugated peoples will retreat only so far. At some point they pick a place where they will fight and die, to preserve not only their honor but their identity.

The underwear was where Sebastian made his stand. To this point he'd been a perfect patient, complying with the countless pokings and proddings, the constant invasion of his privacy, subservience to his lines and his pole, and imprisonment inside 5200. But regressing from underwear to diapers was an indignity he simply would not abide. I tried reasoning, negotiating, and threats. Nothing worked. He cried uncontrollably when I tried to slide a pair of Huggies up his hips; as soon as I had them in place he wiggled violently to pull them off. "I'M A BOY! I'M NOT A BABY!" he yelled.

After two or three failed attempts I acquiesced. Keeping him in underpants would mean changing them every few hours and either throwing the soiled briefs in the garbage or hand-washing them with bleach in the community toilet before cycling them through the shared washer-dryer. Lovely. But if this was to be his only demand, it was worth it. He was worth it.

As the clock wound down to Day 0, the donor unit was undergoing its final prep over at the Cord Blood Bank. Outfitted in lab coats, cryoprotective gloves, and safety glasses, the techs removed the unit from its canister and performed special thawing and washing procedures to awaken the Van Winkled cells from years of slumber at -150° Celsius, tenderly handling the plastic container bag to avoid rupture or contamination. The lab techs hold life in their hands—in cases like ours, the cells weren't just the best match, they were virtually the *only* match. And, as Felicia and I were painfully aware, with cord blood there is no going back for seconds if something goes wrong. This was it.

The donor had a number, not a name: National Marrow Donor Program Unit 9835-7681-1. We knew the donor was male, that he was born before 2010, and that his blood type was O negative. Beyond that, and the fact that he was likely delivered in a North Carolina hospital, nothing. After his precious umbilical cord was donated, the baby could have died in a car crash going home from the hospital; he might have grown up to be the burglar who broke into our apartment; or he could have been the starting forward for the Duke basketball team. According to policy, his family will never be informed the cells were used at all, much less for whom; and we will never meet him. There will be no Emeril Lagasse—hosted moment on live TV.

That part made sense. What I didn't fully comprehend as Dr. Page explained it to me on Day -1 was that, if successful, this transplant would transform our son into a different organism altogether—a person living with *two different kinds of DNA* in his body at once. The cells in Sebastian's skin, hair, and organs would all carry the genes he was born with—the ones Felicia and I gave him—but his blood cells would forever be those of 9835-7681-1. If he were to leave blood at a crime scene, it wouldn't match DNA from a buccal swab of his cheek. (Dr. Page mentioned with an eye roll that TV cop dramas occasionally spin out this little oddity into a plotline.)

The phenomenon is known in medical science as "chimerism," after the mythical Greek beast with the head of a lion, the body of a goat, and the tail of a serpent. In rare instances this occurs naturally, when twin zygotes fuse in the womb to become one. The resulting individual is his or her own twin. Here it happened intentionally—the Duke doctors' business is to create and incubate chimeras to cure deadly disease, and 5200 is, in an industrial sense, a chimera factory—a place where magical creatures are made. It also might be the place where the human species comes closest to playing God. Frankly, it blew my mind—if our son made it through this, he wouldn't be entirely *our* son anymore.

Day -1 was a designated day of rest. The chemo infusions had ended, though the drugs wouldn't fully clear his system for another month. The nurses kicked back Sebastian's diarrhea with yet another medication (loperamide) and he was in good spirits. By now we'd set up additional Thomas train sets on the far side of his bed, so getting anywhere—the bathroom, the fridge, the caregiver's bench/bed—meant tiptoeing through a tangle of intersecting tracks, tunnels, and bridges. In that sense it was just like home.

Felicia had found some published studies suggesting that massage and alternative therapies (aroma, art, and music) help speed recovery during transplant. Using the Connection Room's art supplies, she'd encouraged Sebastian to help color drawings she'd made to depict the process with red markers and glitter glue representing the cells, hoping to boost a mind-body connection that would aid the transplant process or at least make it less scary.

"I need to do all I can to support the healing process in any way his four-year-old brain can understand," she said. That day, she hung the drawings on the wall, telling Sebastian that he was all finished with his "special medicine," and was saying bye-bye to his old cells to make room for New Super Cells. She spent the final hours playing with him, giving him massages with (Prasad-approved) essential oils, and praying.

The weather on Sebastian's rebirthday was glorious. A mild wind, sunny skies, a high of 91. After dropping Lydia off at camp, I headed to 5200, changed and scrubbed, and joined Felicia in the room. After years of anticipation, months of rehabilitation, and weeks of conditioning, this was it—patient and donor unit had both been prepped with microscopic precision for their arranged marriage. All systems were go.

The word "transplant" summons images of a crowded operating room, bloodstained instruments plopping into trays, a surgeon's furrowed brow bespangled with perspiration. When we'd arrived on the Unit I'd assumed the procedure would take place in a designated Transplant Room—a holy of holies with Drs. Prasad and Kurtzberg monitoring every step, a large support staff at the ready should anything go awry.

It turned out to be the most anticlimactic experience of our lives. At 10:30, Nurse Liz and one of her colleagues rolled into the room with a tray of meds and fluids. The donor cells had been transferred to a single, thick infusion syringe that resembled nothing so much as a bottle of Tabasco. Sixty milliliters total; approximately 1.5 billion cells, 100 million per kilo of Sebastian. An ample dose. Kurtzberg had noted the final potency evaluation with enthusiasm on the medical record: "Excellent recovery of progenitor cells post thaw."

But Kurtzberg herself was nowhere to be seen. Neither was Prasad, nor any of the other MDs. The most important medical procedure of Sebastian's life would be performed by the two nurses alone. In fact, this was Liz's first transplant ever. "It's funny because when we go to do transplants, it's like this lifesaving measure, it's what everything's about, and everyone comes in with big thoughts and expectations of what it's supposed to be," she says. "But it's just two nurses doing something that looks just like a blood transfusion. We calculate the drip rate and then find out, based on the size of the unit, how long the doctors want it to go. That's about it."

Prasad wasn't there because, quite simply, he didn't need to be. "The beauty of transplant is not what *we* can do, but what *the cells* can do," he said. "You're infusing them just like IV fluid, and they can take it from there.

"Think of it simply as mechanics. The cells go straight to the heart through the central line, and the heart is pumping one hundred times a minute. Within seconds, the blood you are infusing goes into the rest of the body and gets mixed into the bloodstream. Some cells will get trapped in the spleen and lungs—but there are plenty of them left—and as they pass through the bone marrow, they latch on to it. There is a specific biochemical, molecular connection that causes this. And one by one, the cells jump off the train of the bloodstream and step onto precisely the right platform.

"Because they have this ability, I don't have to do anything. I don't need to stitch anything or repair blood vessels. We just put [the donor unit] in."

The elegant simplicity of the process notwithstanding, success isn't guaranteed. The cells can get off at the right stop but still fail to grow and multiply. And with these cells in particular, the unknowns were compounded. "You can't control how the four out of six match is going to behave inside the body, how the biology is going to play out," one of the doctors said later. "Some things you can control, others you can't. That's where it gets tricky sometimes."

While the power of modern medicine locked horns with the forces of biological entropy inside his body, Sebastian remained serene, oblivious. He required no sedation. He didn't even have to move. He simply sat on his bed playing Fruit Ninja on Felicia's iPhone while the infusion began, a bag of chips at his side. Some kids sleep straight through the whole thing.

Felicia and I held hands and she started to pray. Across the country, many of our friends and family were doing the same. Then it got quiet. The pole took a break from its incessant beeping to honor the occasion. The most fateful moment of our lives took place in near total silence, perturbed only by muted crunches coming from Sebastian's mouth as he devoured his Ruffles.

I was doing something that might be called prayer too. I wasn't petitioning God for a favor, but I was in a state of extreme reverence I'd never felt before. We'd brought our son here, to this place and this moment, the frontier of human and scientific achievement, but the next step, the most important part of the process, the true magic trick, could be performed only by forces beyond the doctors' control. Call it nature, call it the divine, this was the mysterious power to which we now surrendered our son as Abraham did Isaac. Perhaps this power would heal Sebastian; perhaps it could heal our family too. Perhaps, when this was all over, the only word to use would be "miracle."

The nurses kept constant watch on heartbeat and temperature—in rare instances, the infusion can trigger seizures. In those situations, the nurses might pause the process to stabilize the patient, but under no circumstances can the infusion be aborted. This is the one shot, and the doctors' orders are unequivocal—those cells must get into the body by any means necessary.

As the minutes crawled by on hands and knees, a unique smell permeated the room—Sebastian's breath. Prior to storage, the donor cells are treated with a cryoprotectant called DMSO (dimethyl sulfoxide); when they are infused years later, that DMSO works its way into the bloodstream, the lungs, and then out of the body through exhaled air. It smells, strangely, like creamed corn. The scent was funky, and somewhat out of place—it conjured the sense memory of a grade school cafeteria. It was also the smell of success.

It was over in half an hour. The creamed corn smell dissipated; the nurses left. After a light lunch of Oreos with a side of Cool Ranch Doritos, paired with a fine vintage Sprite, Sebastian slid into an afternoon siesta. Felicia rubbed his back and sang softly. I kept my eyes glued to the vital signs monitor above his head, on the lookout for anomalies— true must-see TV.

Happy Rebirthday.

The next morning while flushing the central line, Liz felt a blockage in one of the three lumens. "If you meet resistance, you're not supposed to force it, because the line could pop." She tried clearing it with a declotting solution called heparin, but eventually she concluded there'd been a failure in the central line itself, likely in the plastic mechanism where the three lumens merge into one. The entire line would have to be replaced, which meant an emergency surgery. "At the end of the day, it's equipment," she said with a sigh. "It breaks."

Dr. Prasad was making rounds that morning, and soon entered the little room to give us the "these things happen" speech. Of course, we'd been told to expect many little bumps in the road, but nothing changed the tough truth that Sebastian was about to go under the knife at the precise moment Prasad and Co. had done to his immune system what Rome did to Carthage. "You definitely don't want to put anybody in surgery at Day 1 [the day after transplant]," he later explained, "but looking at the comparative risks, there was no comparison. We needed a fully functioning central line. And we've had to do much more invasive procedures with patients already deep into conditioning. Gallbladder surgeries, bowel resections . . ."

He was right of course, but I was furious nevertheless. This surgery wasn't necessitated by some failing of Sebastian's body—to the contrary, aside from a low potassium level, his body was performing so heroically it deserved its own Marvel movie. No, this was a remedial effort—an extra dose of danger and suffering our son had to endure because the hospital's equipment had failed. Duke was at fault. To my mind, a spectacular snafu like this so early in the journey hadn't happened since Morton-Thiokol installed that defective O-ring on the solid rocket booster that launched the *Challenger*.

As I inhaled to verbalize these thoughts I met Prasad's glance and glimpsed something underneath his imperturbable professional veneer. A hint of vulnerability. The look yanked me out of our immediate situation in Sebastian's tiny room. Consider, said the look, what else is happening on this Unit; the kids and families fighting complications orders of magnitude more severe than Sebastian's. Clara, whose infection and slow engraftment had marooned her on Unit 5200 for ninety days and counting; a girl named Abby Furco, whose GvHD was so severe she'd soon be heading over to the pediatric intensive care unit. Ameena, whom we still hadn't seen outside her room, Allah and fentanyl guiding her through each agonizing hour.

Felicia and I could walk past those rooms, ignorant of the suffering inside, wrapped up in the solipsistic microcosm of our own drama. Prasad could not. Like the other doctors, nurses, and staff on the Unit, when he was on duty he was obliged to enter every room every day, provide world-class professional care with courtesy and compassion, then move on to the next without unloading any of the emotional baggage from the intense encounters he'd just concluded minutes before and a few feet away. The Purell dispenser on the doorway might eradicate the germs from the prior room; nothing can eradicate the emotional intensity of the experience. The fact that the patients are each in a sealed compartment doesn't make their suffering any easier to compartmentalize.

In that moment, Prasad's own pain was visible. "I have moved directly from the room of a leukemia patient who has just relapsed and was heading to hospice, to the room of another patient who's getting discharged in five minutes," he said later. "It's not easy when you're a young resident. You can't just let go of the thought process in one room and move on. Over the years you learn to shut it out, not out of insensitivity but as a responsibility to the individual patient in the next room. You have to be with them one hundred percent, professionally and emotionally, whether you're giving good news or bad."

Dr. Kurtzberg has decades of experience walking the same tightrope. "You kind of learn it on the job. There's no course in medical school called Conveying Bad News. You also have to account for the fact that when you're working with children, you're dealing with their parents, and they might not be in the same place emotionally or share the same knowledge base."

She compares the challenge of making rounds to the challenges of the presidency. "On the same day, the president might be in the Situation Room green-lighting a risky SEAL Team Six mission, then leave to go pardon the Thanksgiving turkey. President Obama could slip back and forth between something intensely serious and something lighthearted. In medicine when you're dealing with very sick patients, you have to do that a lot."

Not every doctor can pull it off. Doctor burnout is a real and costly problem. A 2019 study in the *Annals of Internal Medicine* estimates it drains $4.6 billion from the American health care system every year through medical error, absenteeism, and doctors working less or leaving the field. In a separate study from 2015, 54 percent of doctors (twice the normal rate) reported at least one of the three symptoms of burnout: emotional exhaustion, feelings of cynicism and detachment from work, and a sense of low personal accomplishment.

Different doctors handle the stress differently. Kurtzberg's secret is multitasking. "One thing I do is make sure I have several different things going on, both in the clinic and in the lab," says Kurtzberg. "If you have enough activities going on, some will be going poorly, but others will be going well. It kind of gives you relief from being dragged down into one situation."

Prasad clears his mind with extraprofessional activities. "I play tennis, I'm an amateur photographer, I run on the trails in the Duke forest. And I'm really into cooking," he adds enthusiastically. "I make some really nice kabobs."

Whatever Prasad's Program entailed, it seemed to be underserving him that morning as he laid out the plan for Sebastian's surgery. Something in his affect telegraphed "Please, no attitude today." So I kept my remarks to a minimum and surrendered to reality.

Neither Felicia nor I recall any particulars about the surgery, which happened the next day. Curiously, Sebastian's digital medical records on the Duke My Chart system are remarkably sparse on the matter too. They note an interaction with an anesthesiologist, a chest X-ray, and the delivery of the defective line to the pathology department after its removal. Little else.

Count it as a blessing. It means nothing went wrong. There is little in this world as undervalued as an uneventful day. It would be a month before we saw another.

Chapter 13

HODL
....

In 2013, a cryptocurrency investor posted a now-famous comment on a Bitcoin forum during one of the currency's many violent gyrations. The fat-fingered subject line read: "I AM HODLING!" The term "HODL" has since become crypto slang for the adoption of a patient buy-and-hold strategy in the face of market turmoil. HODL even morphed into an acronym, standing for "Hold on for dear life." As we learned in the weeks after Sebastian's rebirthday, it's a wonderful nonword to live by.

The shitstorm hit with gale force on Day 2. This leg of the journey, as promised, would be the equivalent of rounding Cape Horn.

Two things were happening, both inevitable, both awful. The side effects of the chemo were kicking in; at the same time, Sebastian's body and its new donor cells were trying to sort out their fledging relationship. Flipping the traditional trajectory of a rocky marriage on its head, this couple was expected to *start out* as bitter enemies and over time *end up* as soul mates. These two weeks comprised their fractious honeymoon.

We'd come to a new section on the road map spreadsheet. With conditioning concluded, the columns for the chemo drugs were blank from the boldface Day 0/Transplant row on down.

Three daunting tasks lay ahead, each requiring a Herculean feat of pharmacology. First, avoid infection—for this Nurse Liz and her colleagues began hanging the pole with infusions of an antiviral called acyclovir and an antifungal with which we were intimately familiar after years of usage: voriconazole, referred to by the nurses simply as "the vory." Every two weeks he'd also receive an infusion of immune globulin (IgG) to supply him with antibodies; and every month he'd get an antiprotozoal to ward off lung infection.

Second, keep the rocky marriage intact. Prevent the body from rejecting the transplant and avoid graft-versus-host disease. For this the nurses hung daily doses of two powerful immunosuppressants, CellCept and cyclosporine. These would retard and/or kill any mature T-cells and other lymphocytes that had trickled in from the donor unit during transplant. Such cells would be inclined to attack the host and had to be wiped out.

Third, stimulate the growth of the new cells we *did* want, the fresh lymphocytes and granulocytes hopefully being manufactured from scratch by the donor stem cells now residing in Sebastian's bones. After these new cells were produced they would be trained in the thymus before being released into the system, a gradual process that lasts a hundred days. This needed to happen as rapidly as possible, minimizing the period of the most intense immune vulnerability. To speed things up Sebastian received daily doses of a fascinating drug called filgrastim. Made using recombinant DNA technology, the drug stimulates the bone marrow production of granulocytes (including neutrophils). The drug is officially called G-CSF since it is a granulocyte colony-stimulating factor. In Unit slang, which bestows street names upon many of the important drugs, it's known simply as the G.

In the two-dimensional orthogonal order of the spreadsheet, it all looked so easy to grasp, so reassuring—that's one reason I liked to look at the spreadsheet. In the three-dimensional, flesh-and-blood reality of the room it was another matter. With all the new drugs the pole was now in full bloom, half a dozen infusion pumps affixed round the clock, their respective lights and wires forming a ghastly Christmas tree beside the bed. The rest of the tiny room was in more disarray than a repossessed storage unit—a riot of toys, clothes, books, DVDs, and PlayStation games. Boxes of wipes, sterile gloves, masks, and mouth-rinsing solutions dominated the sink. Add in all the wires, tubes, and equipment and the room felt like the set of a Terry Gilliam movie with blurred boundaries between infrastructure, detritus, and decor. A cluttered cocoon with one purpose: metamorphose a sick kid into a healthy chimera.

In the middle of it all, a child in agony. By Day 2, Sebastian was complaining of intense stomach pain. We knew it was serious when he refused to get out of bed to play trains. He'd been gifted a new locomotive from the Thomas collection, Sir Handel. Normally this would delight Sebastian for hours as he'd learn Sir Handel's personality and work responsibilities, then introduce him to the other dramatis personae arrayed on the tracks. Instead, the treasured toy lay abandoned on the bed.

Then the vomiting began as the mucositis kicked into high gear. The chemo had reduced the top layer of the entire digestive tract to slush. From mouth to anus, all was raw and sore. "The digestive tract is effectively ulcerated through and through," one of the team doctors, Suhag Parikh, explained. It hurt to swallow; it hurt to poop. Looking in Sebastian's ravaged mouth I understood why toothbrushing was forbidden—even a gentle once-over with an Oral-B could have torn his gums into a bloody mess.

As the dead cells pooled in his stomach, its muscles instinctively contracted to eject the irritating contents. The vomit was a gray-green *Ghostbusters* slime. Dr. Parikh later told me that in some cases patients yak up the entire inside lining of their intestine—"It looks like a snake shedding its skin, but from the inside." The imagery is gross; the metaphor apt—the point of the patients' suffering is to shed their anguished pasts. In any event, before things got that grotesque the doctors called for an antinausea med called Zofran; then they began the fentanyl drip. We'd seen our child suffer before; this was the first time his pain was intense enough to require the world's most notorious and addictive opiate.

To no one's surprise, Sebastian stopped eating. Until further notice nutrition would come through the NG tube, if he could keep anything down. He took in enough calories to keep him alive, and not much else. This ordeal would stunt his growth for a year.

A pitiless fever began on Day 4. It hit 105 and stayed there. "We can give Tylenol for the fever," said Dr. Prasad, "but we can't use too much because it can cause liver injury. Over a period of time, it should settle down." Felicia was applying cool compresses on his forehead as we'd always done, but this was different. "As soon as I put a washcloth on his forehead, it gets hot," she texted me. "It's so hard to watch him like this, sedated, just cooking."

A ravenous rash broke out all over his legs, arms, stomach, and neck. Think poison ivy plus sunburn. The doctors ordered a special ointment and cream to keep it in check, but the slimy, Vaselined feeling all over his body only added to his discomfort.

A dry, hacking cough emerged, sending additional waves of pain through his chest and throat with every *heh-ckkkk*. Worse, the breaths between coughs grew raspy and labored. Once again, we had reason to worry about the lungs.

By the end of the day the vital signs monitor was sending up flares—heart rate racing at 220 beats per minute; oxygen saturation levels tumbling from a normal rate in the high 90s down into the 80s, then 70s. They put an oxygen tube in his nose.

This is when the staff's mood shifted from "we just have to ride this out" to bona fide trepidation. It was normal for the early struggles between the graft cells and the host to cause fever and rashes, a phenomenon called engraftment syndrome. It usually subsides over time. But fever is also a classic sign of infection or, as we knew from our misadventures that spring, inflammation-provoked granulomas in CGD patients.

The patient was deteriorating; precise cause unknown. Had Sebastian's pulmonary granuloma outbreak returned? Had he contracted pneumonia? The doctors summoned a bedside X-ray machine for answers. Nurse Liz, usually calm and business-as-usual, came in with the technicians, brow furrowed, hands on hips. "She looked really nervous," Felicia reported later. "She knew that if there was a problem in his lungs, it could be deadly." The team did its work and, leaving Sebastian to his misery, rolled the machine out into the hallway to inspect the image. His fate hung on the results.

Unit 5200 is many things—a hospital, a prison, a community, a retreat. It also sustains comparison to a casino. As we witnessed on Sebastian's rebirthday, the transplant team can control only so much; the rest remains a matter of chance or, for some, divine will. Patients buzzed through the antechamber door on the day of admission cannot know when and in what condition they will leave.

In the darkest hours, the vision of the confetti parade on discharge day buoys the thoughts of patients and families through every blood draw, mouth cleanse, line problem, vomit-splattered bedpan, and befouled undergarment. Imagine—a hallway of nurses, cheerleaders in scrubs and paper booties, applauding and grooving to thumping electropop as their latest Lazarus walks out of the Unit's womb/tomb and out into the light of Healthyworld.

This is no fantasy. A patient can expect to observe or at least overhear a few of these processions during an average stay. The first kid we saw making such a triumphant exit was LeVonna, the infant who'd aced every phase of her transplant, leaving in her mother's arms. The nurses intimated she'd have a tougher life outside the Unit than inside. When I inquired after her years later, no one had any updates, which is generally taken as good news.

A very different kind of departure is rarely discussed and never celebrated. When patients start trending down, their failing organs often require a ventilator or an oscillator, and they are typically transferred to the pediatric intensive care unit. In our nine-page, single-spaced patient treatment plan, the PICU was never once mentioned, much less described, and for good reason. Even for parents who've become inured to the stressors of 5200, the PICU is a shock.

Start with the screaming. The PICU receives patients from car crashes and fires as well as kids struggling with transplant problems or any other type of extreme medical situation. There are no windows, few individual rooms. The space is dominated by the heavy machinery of intensive care—the ventilators and an especially intimidating device for heart and lung support called an ECMO. Together the darkness, the proximity, and the urgency create a "MASH unit," "third world," or "fishbowl" feel, to quote parents who've been there. "Parents say the nurses aren't as friendly," said Nurse Liz, "but that's because they have more responsibility. The PICU nurse treating your kid might have just spent an hour and a half coding another patient to keep them alive, or turned off the respirator to let them die."

"You're watching the nurses go full throttle all the time," said one mom, who watched her daughter go code blue twice, only to be resuscitated each time by the scrambling staff. "It makes for some pretty intense conversations."

"Everything you have that makes you feel safe on the PBMTU gets stripped away in a second," said another mom, who'd spent a week there with her daughter on a respirator. There are reasons to be scared—the stats are grim. Duke clinical social worker Lindsay Gallo estimates that 40 percent of the transplant kids who move to the PICU don't make it out alive. "I watched a lot of kids roll past our room on the way over there," said one mother who spent months on 5200. "I didn't see many of those kids roll back."

The PICU entered our conversation the moment Sebastian's breathing became an issue. If his breathing kept getting worse, Prasad explained, he'd be heading to the PICU for ventilation.

Prasad picked his words carefully, making clear that it wasn't so out of the ordinary, trying to make us comfortable with what was clearly a worst-case scenario. "We are hoping he doesn't need to go, but if so it would only be for a few days to give his lungs a little boost. Okaayyy?"

As Felicia and I stood over our child, watching his escalating anguish, the consequences of our decision sank in. He was paying the price for the path we'd picked for him, the fully ablative chemotherapy the Duke doctors had laid out in his treatment plan. And the point I need to make is this: we had it easy.

Repeating for emphasis: we had it easy.

Years later, in an emotional conversation I had with her mother, Amanda Assell, I learned the details of what happened with Khaleda, who'd died while the Assells were staying next door to us at the Alden Place apartments. Amanda had blogged beautifully during their experience, composing a soaring obituary of the short but inspiring life of a girl who dreamed of weddings and whose last dying wish was to have a simple dinner with her family. I wanted to know more details about their experience on the Unit, and Amanda was kind enough to share.

As mentioned earlier, Khaleda had survived fourteen years with beta-thalassemia major, a feat all the more impressive given that the first seven of those years were spent in Kabul, one of the toughest places on earth to be seriously sick. Amanda and her husband, Mike, adopted her and spent years and countless dollars getting her the complex treatment required just to get her healthy enough to survive a transplant. Khaleda caught a break when one of her brothers back in Afghanistan tested as a perfect match, and they went into 5200 just before Thanksgiving 2015, expecting to be discharged in forty-five days.

Like us, the Assells had read and signed off on all the potential complications from the chemo. Unlike us, their daughter had to endure most of them. For some reason, Khaleda's body metabolized the chemo drugs much slower than anticipated; the toxins stayed in her system too long, wreaking havoc on her organs, and she suffered the equivalent of a massive overdose. The doctors had to dial back and eventually discontinue the conditioning to keep from killing her on the spot.

Perhaps that would have been better. The ensuing side effects included a nearly lethal bladder problem, blood clots, severe mucositis, VOD in the liver, a lung infection. Khaleda spent a week in the PICU and on a ventilator for a week; she spent months back on the Unit with all sorts of tubes inside her. "Three of the doctors who'd worked together for twenty years said the suffering she went through was as much as they'd ever seen," said Amanda. "What we watched happen... it was shocking that the human body could withstand it. But she never complained."

Tragically, it was all for naught. The interruption of the conditioning meant Khaleda's existing immune system hadn't been entirely eradicated. Post-transplant, it resurged and wiped out the donor cells. The transplant failed. After a staggering 170 days on the Unit, her oxygen levels descending, Khaleda called her family and her primary nurse to her bedside. She drifted in and out of consciousness for a few hours while they prayed and said goodbye. She died peacefully at 10:30 in the morning.

Allowing a patient to die with dignity may seem like a no-brainer, but a senior nurse named Bobbie Caraher, who'd earned her stripes working in war-zone refugee camps, says she had to fight for years to get the transplanters to recognize there comes a time when their sorcery can work no more wonders, a time to let the patient go. "The culture of the Unit used to be 'We're going to save you, everyone has to survive,'" she told me. "Some doctors didn't want to give the families bad news and admit defeat, even if it meant keeping a patient on life support in the PICU for months. It wasn't fair." Now, thanks in part to Bobbie's persistence, palliative and hospice teams get involved when it's clear a patient isn't going to make it.

Fortunately, that's a rarity. The Assells' experience was extreme, and it would be irresponsible to suggest it was in any way representative. Much more typical is the experience of Lilly Hicks, a teenage leukemia patient who was one of Sebastian's neighbors on the Unit. Today she's a happy teenager navigating eleventh grade back home in Greensboro.

But even the successful ones often have grueling complications. On Sebastian's second week post-transplant, just as he was at his worst, we saw Justine Richels and baby Thor in the hallway. This was unexpected—they were supposed to be long gone. Aside from a disturbing episode where Thor had taken too much fentanyl and momentarily stopped breathing (it's notoriously tough to administer perfect dosages for kids that small), the kid had rocked his transplant and enjoyed his confetti parade two months before—an inspiration for the rest of us.

Now he was back, and his parents' wide smiles had vanished. The day before his scheduled return to Minnesota, Thor's final ultrasound had turned up a large puddle of fluid buildup in his chest. His heart was floating in it. Prasad called them back to 5200 immediately and ordered a surgery to drain Thor's chest cavity. Twelve ounces of fluid poured out of the eighteen-month-old's thorax, and it didn't stop there. Thor required a drainage tube that ran from the pericardial sac, through the ribs, and out the side of his body before the problem was fixed. That took a month.

At least CGD patients like Thor who endured tough setbacks could cling to the knowledge that a successful transplant would be a complete cure. Many patients we met had conditions a transplant could only ameliorate or decelerate. At night when I couldn't sleep I'd walk the hall and peek into the doctor's room, where the overnight attending usually sits at the conference table reviewing records, awaiting the next crisis. On the far wall a large whiteboard charts each room, patient, type of transplant, and their original disease, among other data. I'd been immersed in the world of rare genetic disorders for four years and I was still bewildered by half the conditions listed. Batten disease, Hurler syndrome, other three-letter acronyms I can't recall—cruel, relentless disorders that typically condemn patients to abbreviated and sorrowful lives. The patients and their families endure all the travails of transplant without any hope of ever putting their diseases completely behind them. The best they can hope for is a marginal improvement in quality and/or quantity of life. Yet despite that discouraging risk/reward ratio, here they were, cooking pasta in the kitchen, making buttons in the Connection Room, bravely sticking it out and moving through their tunnel toward the light, no matter how faint or flickering it may be.

Were all the parents saints? Far from it. As I knew firsthand, sometimes we rose to the occasion, sometimes we sank below it.

"There's a strong chance you're going to lose it at least once while you're here," a social worker had said back when we first arrived. "We put you in a pressure cooker. You may explode."

"I've had parents say, 'I'm done, we're leaving' right in the middle of transplant," said Gallo. "They don't mean that, but they are emotionally and physically exhausted. They feel like they can't continue." And if things go south for the kids, despair can turn to anger. One of the moms on the Unit during our stay even got violent with the nurses. "She had a really bad temper," one nurse told me. "She would lose it and start swinging at the staff. We had to call security. That was a very serious case."

That mother was almost barred from the Unit during her own daughter's transplant. And while those crazy situations are rare, low-grade breakdowns and outbursts are not. "Most of the time families will say afterward that it was harder than they'd thought it would be," said Gallo. "Rarely do families say it was easier."

Felicia peered through the venetian blinds, reading the consternation on Nurse Liz's face as the radiologist and Dr. Prasad reviewed the chest X-ray. A minute later Liz broke into a broad smile, her whole body relaxing as she looked at Felicia through the window and gave a thumbs-up. The lungs were clear. "Our little man's doing really good."

Later that day Prasad came in by himself while Felicia was in the room. "He went to the computer and modified something. He looked concerned and said we need to keep monitoring Sebastian closely, but it looked like things were going in the right direction."

Felicia had no questions. "Sometimes there's nothing more to say. There was nothing more that he knew or that I needed to know."

When Felicia was on duty, she leaned heavily on the alternative therapies to get Sebastian through each hour. She'd give him foot and back rubs with essential oils; she'd play his favorite songs and sing along (the humongous Hawaiian ukulele singer's version of "Somewhere Over the Rainbow" was a favorite); and like so many other moms on the Unit, she prayed. "I can't describe it and I don't expect you to understand," she told me, "but here in this place, I feel a connection to God."

For a few of those desperate days, while Sebastian's head was still hot as a cauldron, I was called back to New York for work. One of Felicia's church group friends came to relieve her, reassuring her with a smile as she took over washcloth duty. Another angel.

Felicia spent some of that precious downtime in the hospital's nondenominational chapel/meditation space. There was a large book there, opened and placed on a pedestal—not a sacred text but a public comments book in which families shared thoughts and stories. Felicia made it a regular practice to stop by, both to write her own remarks and read others'. "I find strength from the writings of the families," she told me. "They make me feel that I'm not alone; that I am not weird for having these feelings about God."

She ran her fingers over the words on the pages, as if to connect to the hope within them. She felt as if she were praying along with these families, tapping into a source of divine support. This was a prime example of John Dominic Crossan's metaphor of God as an airport courtesy outlet. Fully recharged, Felicia could return to the Unit with the strength to forge ahead.

When I returned, I tried to manage things during my shifts like a TV producer—that is, with Prussian efficiency. I kept Sebastian's mental state out of a downward spiral using the same methods I deployed on myself—focusing on the proper and prompt execution of the next item on the to-do list. Now we pee, now we drink, now we barf, now we wash the mouth, now we bathe. Any discrete activity, no matter how tedious or routine, can be framed as a step forward.

I also tried the Patch Adams thing. The easiest part was just being silly—stupid fart noises were part of my standard repertoire; I'd also regularly take on the persona of a magician or conjurer and, calling upon some presumed collective sentience of the donor cells, command them to "GROWWWW . . . and MUULITPLYYYY." He got a kick out of that.

Then I'd tell some actual joke jokes. He didn't get them, but he knew enough about the mechanics and etiquette of comedy to know that after the teller delivers the punch line, the listener is supposed to laugh, so he obliged.

Here's one from Rodney Dangerfield he eventually learned by heart: "A guy goes to the doctor; doctor tells him, 'Ya got cancer.' The guy says, 'I want a second opinion.' Doctor says, 'Okay . . . You're ugly too!'"

My standup routine, however effective, was but a warm-up act for the great entertainer, Sebastian's sister. Lydia could only spend a few hours on the Unit at a time, but each of her visits was rocket fuel for her brother's spirits. There were days when Sebastian looked worse than Mimi at the end of *La Bohème*, curled up in his bed, miserable and counting the minutes till he could press the button for a fentanyl hit (to avoid opioid addiction, the patient is only allowed one small dose every twenty minutes). Then Lydia would bound into the room and he'd spring to life and hop down on the floor to play trains, as if the whole "sick thing" were just a ploy for attention. And if she was there to encourage him, he'd summon the strength and humility to visit the Connection Room with his despised pole in tow. There were shelves full of games and crafts, and volunteers to wipe them all down after every use. For the better part of an hour, he was almost his old self.

Nights were much longer and much harder. He'd wake up at odd hours, nauseous, febrile, shaking, coughing, weeping. To calm him I'd put on the local classical music station; he found it soothing enough that eventually he'd request it. At 2 a.m. on Day 11, I remember holding his hot little body, rocking back and forth on the bed in the dark as tears streamed down our respective cheeks while Itzhak Perlman played Bach's Violin Sonata no. 1.

Sebastian hit rock bottom two days later when the force of his cough ruptured the capillaries in his eyes. He had no platelets to retard bleeding; 80 percent of his corneas turned dark red. The doctors said his vision was fine and the eyes would clear eventually. "Sometimes the low platelets can cause rare complications, major bleeding in the brain or the abdomen," said Prasad, "but that risk is very small because we are so proactive monitoring the count." Still, our son looked like he'd just survived a gang initiation. This was the closest we came to losing it.

Sebastian's ability to HODL was perhaps his greatest gift. By Day 16, his fever receded to 102 and he regained the strength to walk laps in the hall. I took him to the laminated "Today I Feel . . ." poster, and without pause he raised his atrophied arm in silence and pointed to the impossibly wide smile on the face above the word "ECSTATIC."

His eyes were filled with blood but devoid of fear. This four-year-old child had stared down the angel of death once more, and he was prepared to HODL through whatever the Unit would throw at him next. It was the greatest privilege of our lives to be at his side.

Chapter 14

Engraftment

....

The liberation of Raqqa was proceeding with alacrity. Brandishing a sawed-off Mossberg in my left hand and Excalibur in my right, I'd maintained an 80 percent kill ratio as we pushed up from our landing zone on the north bank of the Euphrates past the Syria International Islamic Bank. The makeshift prison compound was in the old amusement park and as I approached its perimeter I leapt in slow motion over a row of white Toyota Land Cruisers, the must-have ISIS-mobile. From fifteen feet in the air I plopped a grenade onto the keffiyeh of the caliphate commander in charge. Bull's-eye. It detonated just as I landed on the far side of a courtyard, the grass ground to dirt, and snapped the hyoid bone of a dumbstruck jihadi blocking the door of a one-story cinder-block building. Inside, across the dusty floor, I found the hostage huddled over a cold bowl of rice, her shackled hands clutching a wooden spoon. I put down the shotgun to take off her niqab. This time she was Elizabeth Taylor from *A Place in the Sun*. I cut her loose with the sword and we scrambled out the back to discover my 1974 Oldsmobile 98 Regency—the first car I'd ever owned—parked next to a commandeered Iraqi tank. The Olds' red ignition key appeared in my hand and we eased in, backed out, and tore off. Over my headset the other members of my unit—Allen Iverson, Clint Eastwood, and Garry Kasparov—told me I was "da man." Liz leaned in for a kiss. I plunged into her violet eyes. From the sky there came a beeping noise. Then I woke up.

It was midnight on 5200. Despite the late hour, medical doings were afoot. The pole was doing its best R2-D2.The night shift nurse entered the room to appease it, take Sebastian's vitals, and draw blood. Whatever dream state fentanyl transports one to, he was still there.

I sat up, the flesh on my arm making the familiar *prrffft* sound as it peeled off the upholstery. Transitioning from my dream to this reality was always a profound bummer, and I tried to ward off despair with a quickie two-minute meditation. Rebooted, the brain went back on duty—MUST KEEP BOY ALIVE.

The umpteenth quirk of life on the Unit: the wee hours often provide the highlight of the day. The staff is a fraction of the day shift's, the patients are usually asleep, and there are no visitors; but this is the magic hour when the daily blood work numbers come back from the lab. As I affixed a hiker's headlamp to my forehead to read a little Vonnegut, someone in a white coat was looking through a microscope and manually counting the cells on a slide of Sebastian's blood. At this stage of the process, there was nothing on earth more important than those numbers.

By this point we were thirsty with anticipation as we awaited the next make-or-break step of the transplant process: engraftment. This milestone was the official confirmation that the donor cells had nestled into their new home in Sebastian's bones and begun making enough fresh new cells that they were venturing into the bloodstream in numbers noticeable enough to count. The chemo had taken the old bad cells from normal levels down to zero; now the new cells, aided by the G, had to climb back up from zero to normal. This was the skeleton key to the door standing between Sebastian's painful past and a future as open as the night sky.

"Engraftment"—sometimes, when I said the word low and slow in the timbre of the voiceover guy who does those "In a wurrrld" movie trailers, it sounded like a Crichton techno-thriller. When Prasad said it with the plosives of his Indian accent, it sounded like a spell from Dungeons & Dragons. But the formal announcement of engraftment would most likely be made in the honey-tongued Carolina drawl of a night nurse, reading little numbers on the lab results. Success meant we could advance to the next level of this video game; failure meant returning to square one—the search for another donor unit; more chemo; another rebirthday; another trip around the Horn with the side effects and engraftment syndrome. And the sequel would have only a 50 percent chance of a happy ending.

It wouldn't happen all at once. Engraftment is defined as three consecutive days when the blood's absolute neutrophil count (ANC) rises above 500. The ANC, in turn, is calculated from the blood work delivered by the lab each night. For the patients on the Unit awaiting the good news, the stroke of twelve can be as joyous as New Year's Eve.

The length of the wait varies wildly—some patients zip through and engraft within two weeks; others take three months or more. In many cases the ANC crosses 500 for 24 gleeful hours, only to sink back down again, adding to the suspense and sometimes the heartbreak. "It's super-individualized," said Nurse Liz. "There's no rhyme or reason. Parents want to know how long it should take, it's one of the questions we get a lot; and we always have the same pat answer: 'It just depends...' which everyone hates to hear, but it's true."

When engraftment finally arrives, it's always cause for celebration. The nurses mark the moment by creating large custom posters for the patient, which we'd seen hanging on the doors of the lucky patients' rooms. (The artsy-craftsy aspect of life on 5200 engrosses staff as well as patients.) Sebastian's neighbors Ameena and Lilly already had their posters—Lilly's featured a large tree and a construction paper sun with three owls, each displaying the ANC counts from the first three days over 500. LILLY ENGRAFTED! read the block letters. As much as any diploma or trophy could ever be, these posters were a testament to the achievement of the child and the dedication of the parents.

We wanted one.

It was still too early to expect much progress. Nevertheless, in a spasm of optimism, I walked out to the nurses' station to await the labs. They came back as expected: Sebastian's white blood cell counts were still bouncing off the bottom. The power of the G notwithstanding, there was nothing to do but wait; keep the kid alive; and watch closely, extremely closely. When the patients are so immunocompromised, their vulnerability to infection means things can fall apart within hours. "You might walk in on a patient who's had a really good stable day, then all of a sudden their stats drop overnight," Liz said. "Kids can hold their vitals for a long time, but once they can't, it's almost an instantaneous response. They decompose much faster than adults." I'd caught a brief glimpse of what she meant the previous week when one of the kids coded shortly after the 9 p.m. lights-out. The entire staff went running down the hall. I didn't know precisely what happened, and I didn't want to.

I stopped in the parents' bathroom on the way back to Sebastian's bedside. After I disinfected every surface, I examined myself in the mirror. A few days' stubble and bloodshot eyes laid the foundation for the Atlantic City grifter look I'd been cultivating since our arrival. I lowered my chin and examined my scalp—I was losing hair faster than my chemo-soaked son. The mucocele inside my lower lip was still there, and I was tonguing it more than ever. As I massaged my expanding muffin top I thought wistfully of the treadmill I'd discovered in the Unit's supply room when Sebastian had first been admitted. Determined to emerge victorious and unbroken from this place, I'd envisioned pounding out three miles every morning before breakfast.

But the motor on the thing was blown and I hadn't worked out in weeks. Meanwhile my caloric intake, as usual determined largely by the content of my children's leftovers, had been drawn into the orbit of Sebastian's aforementioned junk food diet. The results were already noticeable—my man boobs were growing, as was my preference for elastic waistbands. Repulsed, I shuffled back to the room, resolving to avoid all cameras and reflective surfaces until further notice.

Felicia once remarked, in a tone at once complimentary and pejorative, that I was the kind of guy who would do well in prison. She was referring to my ability to keep myself occupied for extended periods with solitary pursuits such as reading, chess, piano, and television. I'd been honing that skill nonstop during our tenure on the Unit. As I tried to settle back onto the couch bed, I indulged a destructive habit of fiddling on my iPhone. I chewed up the next two hours checking off-season NFL news, burrowing down YouTube rabbit holes, and sniffing around the Facebook pages of long-lost friends I'd almost certainly never see again in person. Whatever dopamine fix the phone supplied, it was no substitute for sleep.

Dr. Stephanie Cacioppo, an assistant professor of psychiatry and behavioral neuroscience at the University of Chicago, ties social isolation to diminished hippocampus function in the brain, resulting in memory loss, cognitive decline, and depression. After a month of isolation, according to one study, neurons in sensory and motor regions of the brain shrink by 20 percent. Cacioppo is one of a growing number of scientists who oppose solitary confinement in prisons; some of the ex-cons they've studied lost their ability to navigate or recognize faces, at least temporarily.

Interestingly, Cacioppo believes connection to a larger group or higher purpose supplies the brain a degree of resilience in such environments: "Collective identity is protective against individual loneliness." We had a collective identity in abundance—the solidarity with the other families on the Unit and with the many other patient families in and around the hospital.

Felicia regularly found that solidarity in the hospital chapel, and before she arrived that morning to relieve me, Felicia swung by there to prepare for the day ahead. On the most recent pages of the public comments book, she noticed that some of the writers who'd written prayers during their toughest times had returned later, after their loved one had healed, to give God thanks. She silently hoped she could soon do the same.

For now, she made the following entry: "This process is an opportunity to become who we are meant to be, so we're not so burdened with the fear, the anger. I remain convinced that through suffering we grow, and through intense suffering we grow further."

Spiritually fortified, Felicia scrubbed on to the Unit at 9 a.m., after Sebastian had completed his morning ablutions. We had one of our typical status update conversations. Straining to sound medically fluent, I tried to channel Prasad while she did her best Kurtzberg.

"It looks like we're past the worst engraftment syndrome symptoms," I began. "No barfing last night, the fever is inching down, and the vitals are back to normal."

"The cough?"

"On and off. Wasn't bad enough to keep him up."

"Did he eat anything?"

"No, still through the tube only."

"The rash?"

"Put on cream at bedtime and after the labs came back. The attending checked it this morning and said it's getting better."

"So he's not in pain?"

"Certainly not as much."

"Good. Can we talk to them about getting off the fentanyl?"

"Yeah, you should ask about that." We knew the fentanyl couldn't just stop—the doctors wean the kids off gradually to prevent opioid withdrawal.

I departed as Felicia retrieved a drawing pad and markers from the plastic bins in the corner, sat down on the bed, and began to sketch a happy family holding hands with a rainbow. Those were the images she wanted Sebastian to focus on.

"*Growwwww . . . and multiplyyy*," I commanded the cells as I left.

As the days trickled by, the daily ANC began creeping slowly toward the 500 mark—126, 162, 192. On June 30, it jumped to 418, only to slide back to 414 on July 1. By now we'd become accustomed to the good news/bad news pendulum of life on the Unit. "It's super disappointing," Liz said, "but it happens quite often. Remember, the manual count is just capturing a snapshot of the cells, recording whatever they are doing at that time. It fluctuates by the hour."

When not attending to her official duties, Liz was working on a special secret project in the nurses' lounge—she'd begun Sebastian's engraftment poster. "Some nurses are superstitious and won't start until they see the numbers for engraftment on that third day, but I just had a feeling."

Liz didn't share this with us during the darkest hours of the previous weeks, but while Sebastian was *in extremis* she'd interpreted all his hideous symptoms as good signs. They meant things were going according to plan. Had the engraftment syndrome not appeared, it would have meant engraftment wasn't happening at all, which would have been much worse. "With the fevers, the vomiting, the rash, he'd pretty much checked every box," Liz recalled. "Once we ruled out lung infection, it meant he was in a bad place, but we were going to get to a good place. And when I saw him turn the corner, I knew we were going to see the numbers changing."

Still, she didn't want to get us excited prematurely. She made sure we didn't catch her at the nurses' station furtively cutting out paper loco-motives and tracks between the cyclosporine and CellCept hangs. She'd known the design concept from Day -14. "Clearly it was going to be *Thomas & Friends;* some kids will want *PAW Patrol* one day, then *Frozen,* then something else. But with Sebastian it was easy."

I was wrapping up a Michael Caine movie marathon alone in the communal Caregiver Room when the results came in at 2 a.m. on July 2. ANC = 516. I texted Felicia the good news so she'd see it first thing when she woke up back at the Alden Place apartment, then walked into Sebastian's room. Felicia had draped the pole with a little blue polyes-ter Superman cape, and as it stood silent guard over my sleeping son, I recognized it for the first time as the hero it was—defender, nourisher, resurrector. His own metal Yggdrasil, a bridge from past to future.

Inside his body, a silent symphony of biology and medicine was in its *vivace* movement. The lymphocyte suppressants; the antiviral, anti-fungal, and antibiotic prophylaxis, the IgG supplement; the liver-protecting Actigall; the nutrition fed through the NG tube—all playing their parts so that the new donor cells, amplified by the dazzling power of the G, could make their glorious debut.

Bring it on.

July 3, Lydia's eighth birthday, saw the ANC jump to 605. Two straight days over 500—we were on the brink of a breakthrough.

We'd arranged a birthday party for Lydia at a local rock-climbing place. Tina Merrill came with her son, Sam; Hunter Glass with his daughter, Sammie. We spent the late afternoon at the Alden Place pool, the kids enjoying some chlorinated fun while Hunter sunbathed and cracked nonstop on Hillary Clinton. I returned to 5200 late that night with a slice of Lydia's birthday cake—a red velvet number that, for no particular reason, she'd asked to be decorated with the baker's best forgery of Van Gogh's *Starry Night.* The cake looked better than it tasted, but Sebastian eagerly swallowed several bites, his first solid food in weeks.

That evening I perused the latest issue of the Unit's glossy monthly newsletter, *The Community Counts*. In its perpetually positive prose, it highlighted recent happenings on the Unit with happy snaps of the masked patients playing in the activity room, a successful fundraising golf tournament, the comings and goings of beloved staffers, and up-lifting testimonials from post-transplant patients with news of their restored lives and boundless gratitude. Sebastian was one of the kids featured in the regular "New Kids on the Block" section, and as I held up the color photo of him in the upper-right corner of the page I com-pared the smiling pre-transplant face I saw there to the swollen, NG-tubed, balding, bloodshot one in the bed. It was scarcely recognizable. *We have done this to our child,* I thought, *and we may never see his old face again.*

Then he grinned and asked to hear the Rodney Dangerfield joke: "So, a guy goes to the doctor . . ."

That night I could feel it coming like Phil Collins. If memory serves, the duty nurse was Jenna Boyd, a sunny twenty-five-year-old from Raleigh who looked young enough to fit in with the cheerleaders at a Duke basketball game. She was a deeply serious young woman who'd grown up with a severely autistic sister and had devoted her life to helping children. I wanted to be awake when the labs came in. I was on the couch bed with my chess app, trying to memorize variations of the Caro-Kann Defense, when she entered with the news: ANC = 540.

My text to Felicia was more of a telegram.

ANC 540. Engraftment. He did it. I love you.

There was nothing more to say.

It was the Fourth of July and as Felicia entered the room with Lydia the next day, she busted out a bag of red, white, and blue streamers, noisemakers, an Uncle Sam hat, and other patriotic party favors. As unbridled exuberance is not really my thing, I stood and smiled while the three of them grooved and sang along with Taio Cruz's "Dynamite" chirping out of Felicia's iPhone. Sebastian waved the flag.

Prasad came by to congratulate us. I remembered him saying he'd been involved in three thousand transplants over the course of his career. "Now you can say three thousand and one!" I joked. It was the first and last time I cracked him up.

An hour later it was party time out in the hall. The Unit staff seizes any excuse to get the kids out of their beds; the Fourth of July is always a biggie. The hallway reverberated with the sounds of Sousa, and confetti filled the air as a little patients' parade kicked off. The kids confined to wheelchairs and walkers led the way. Then the infants, like baby Thor, cradled in their mothers' arms. Ambulatory patients like our neighbor Lilly, who'd been honored as a "Super Stepper" in the monthly newsletter for her lap-walking prowess, brought up the rear—the mask could not hide her twinkling eyes. And, tailing the procession, Lydia—a plenipotentiary for her brother and the other kids who couldn't leave their rooms. The procession started outside the caregivers' room. The marchers turned left at the nurses' station, walked past the exit door they might or might not ever pass through, and stopped at the other end of the hall past the supply room. The walk was eighty yards max, but it was the most inspiring act of pedestrian courage I'd seen since the end of On the Waterfront.

When we returned to the room, Nurse Liz had affixed the engraftment poster to the wall. Thomas beamed forth, flanked by his friends Percy and James, the puffs of smoke from their respective funnels proclaiming: July 2, ANC 516; July 3, ANC 605; July 4, ANC 540. SEBASTIAN ENGRAFTED! blared the block letters as fireworks exploded in the background.

Later that afternoon, Lydia, bursting with joy, joined other siblings as they drew window art with large grease pencils in the hallway outside, a traditional part of the Unit's art therapy program. Her window portrayed a series of fireworks exploding above a little boy in a boat.

"Mommy, do you like my artwork?" she asked Felicia, her eyes glowing with delight. "Can you see the little boy in the boat? That's Sebastian, Mom! He's watching the fireworks!"

Later that night he saw the real thing. After petitioning the doctors for special permission, Nurse Liz got Sebastian his first furlough outside the Unit—for one hour and not a minute longer. At twilight, we disconnected the pole and loaded him into one of the Unit's red wagons. Liz guided the four of us out through the antechamber doors and onto a special elevator that took us to the rooftop helipad used by the Duke Life Flight team. The crew had gathered there to greet us and show the kids around the chopper (once we'd Clorox-wiped the interior).

As dusk turned to night, fireworks displays around the Raleigh-Durham area bloomed along the horizon. Sebastian, his face shielded by a mask, was taking his first breaths of freedom—from the confinements of his hospital room and his disease—on Independence Day. In the sticky summer air, Felicia and I caught the whiff of a future in which our son would hold our hands as we died contentedly, not the tragic converse.

Cure the kid, cure the marriage, cure the soul, live happily ever after. A great chain reaction of healing played out in our imaginations. But constructing narratives out of desires is a dangerous thing. The forces of chaos still govern more of life than any of us can fully accept. On the helipad that night, the Life Flight crew looked as strong, skilled, and evolved as any prime specimen of the human race, especially compared to the enfeebled transplant kid sitting in their chopper. And yet, three of them, along with a cancer patient they were transporting, would lose their lives in an instant when that same chopper crashed the following year. We wept when we heard the news; the universe shrugged its shoulders. Khaleda's mourning mother, Amanda Assell, said it best: "We assume life is going to go a certain way and we'll all live to a happy old age. But that's just not how everybody's life goes. Tomorrow is not promised."

Chapter 15

Get Out

....

Roll a pair of dice twenty times. The odds of coming up snake eyes on any given roll—one in thirty-six—never change. Each instance is an exercise in unconditioned probability. And yet, if you've gone fifteen, sixteen, seventeen times without hitting it once, it's natural, if irrational, to suspect you're increasingly likely to hit double ones with each successive roll. The mind convinces itself it's due for some bad luck—a textbook case of superstitious thinking.

Though Unit 5200 is ruled by the unbending discipline of scientific reasoning, superstitious thinking can infiltrate a patient's room like any virus. For those inclined to worry, each trouble-free day brings an incrementally stronger suspicion of an impending reversal. The dice-rolling comparison isn't entirely congruous, as a patient's condition today is plainly connected to his/her condition yesterday—these aren't independent dice rolls—but that only makes the superstition all the more irrational. If you've gone ten straight days on the Unit with no complications, the odds of having one on the eleventh are likely *lower* than before; yet the tendency is to believe they are *higher.*

To minimize the corrosive effect of such thinking, we tried to stay focused on hitting the next milestone. After engraftment, that goal was simple: *get out.* Build up the patient's cell count, blood chemistry, caloric intake, weight, and other stats to such impressive levels the doctors are willing to release the child back to his/her local lodgings. The kid still won't be allowed to go *home* home for months, movement will still be severely restricted, and daily visits to the Valvano Day Hospital are a must. But at least the patient can go back to living with family, eating and sleeping like a normal person, and begin the pains-taking process of reintegrating into Healthyworld. A worthy prize.

To make it to his confetti parade and out the exit door, Sebastian had to build up his cell counts and strength. To that end, we kept him on a firm schedule of hallway walks. If he didn't want to be seen in public with his pole I'd make him jump up and down on his bed—the nurses said exercise of any kind stimulates cell production.

Felicia also continued with regular foot rubs. She'd taken a fancy to reflexology, and assured me it was helping. "The nerves of the foot connect to the heart and the lungs," she advised.

"Okaaayyy," I replied in my best Prasad voice. "Can't hurt."

While focusing on his progress, Sebastian also had to remain infec-tion free. Despite engraftment, his innate immune system was still nascent, and his acquired immune system would take a full year or more to mature. Given all the precautions on the Unit, infection seemed unlikely. Yet the pathogens still broke through those defenses with startling frequency, wreaking havoc on hopeful families. Just down the hall, Clara had come down with the *C. diff* bacteria; it halted her progress and confined her to her room for months. We later met a teenage girl who contracted a wicked case of cytomegalovirus that, among other things, attacked her retina. She spent an extra *year* in Durham in and out of the Unit. And up at NIH, Dr. Malech told us of a tragic case of a CGD patient who died at the NIH post-transplant after contracting the dreaded MRSA that resists most antibiotics. Unfortunately, hospital-acquired infection remains a real problem even at top facilities, resulting in thousands of U.S. deaths each year. Every day on the Unit was a risk.

The second ongoing threat was graft-versus-host disease, which often pops up long after engraftment. If the uneasy marriage between donor cells and Sebastian's body degenerated into full-blown war, the result could be gruesome. We'd seen what GvHD could do—Abby Furco, the girl who was sent to PICU and later hospice care, had a wicked case—her kidneys were torn up and her skin developed a rash so angry she looked like she had third-degree burns on her arms and face as she'd marched bravely in the Unit's Independence Day parade. Even Lilly, our neighbor on the Unit and the resident record holder for fastest engraftment, caught a mild case of GvHD in her GI tract and required an endoscopy. "She was vomiting up stuff that looked like it came from Middle Earth," said her father. When it got ugly, her mom went into the bathroom so Lilly wouldn't see her cry.

Fortunately, Kurtzberg reminded us, severe or chronic GvHD is rare in cord blood transplants. "The donor cells from umbilical cords are so naive and malleable they have an easier time getting along with their hosts," she said. This was the grand bargain for her CGD protocol—harsher chemo, but lower odds of GvHD.

We still had to worry about the reverse scenario—the host attacking the graft. Sometimes a patient's body will kill off the donor cells, rendering the entire transplant a failure. I was perplexed to hear this was still a possibility post-engraftment, especially since on the surface, Sebastian's blood counts looked better with each passing day. On July 5, the ANC shot up to 1,012, nearly doubling overnight. The daily doses of the G were paying dividends. Over the next several days some of his charts resembled the hockey stick stock charts of a hot IPO.

"How can the transplant still fail with numbers like these?" I asked

Dr. Martin during the week it was his turn to make the morning rounds. "Aren't these manual blood counts proof that new white cells are pouring into the bloodstream?"

"Yes," he explained patiently, "but we didn't yet know for sure whether these new cells are coming from *good* new donor cells or *bad* old CGD cells."

In other words, we couldn't completely trust the 0.0 readings we'd seen in the first postchemo blood counts—there was still a chance the chemo carpet-bombing hadn't completely eradicated the old cells. For all we knew, the lab tech who provided the great news about the rising ANC weeks later could have been observing cells spawned from the original, deficient immune system. The whole engraftment celebration could have been a cruel joke.

We wouldn't be sure that the new cells, which had prompted so much rejoicing, were really the right kind until we saw the results of a genetic inspection—a chimerism test—scheduled for Day 26. Dr. Kurtzberg had warned us that chimerism is harder to achieve in CGD patients—the original immune system is hard to knock out, which is why the chemo needed to be so harsh. At the same time, Dr. Prasad had given Sebastian a 90 percent chance of making it. Given the track record of the Duke protocol, a failed transplant would be highly unusual.

And yet, for rare-disease families, the highly unusual has a nasty habit of popping up unexpectedly. As I write this section, a CGD family at Duke is reeling from the news that their son's transplant failed in precisely this manner. Their Facebook post from Day 40, eleven days after they'd experienced the joy of engraftment, is devastating: "We are shocked. We are terrified. We are broken. . . . How can we celebrate any positive results going forward when every time we get good news, it's followed by bad news? . . . What do we have to do to catch a break? What kind of test is this, God? Hasn't [our son] suffered enough?"

As I write the second draft, they are mourning his death.

It was a period of departures and arrivals. The Unit is not like camp or school—you don't graduate simultaneously with your class. Lilly had her confetti parade and headed back to the Ronald McDonald House. Ameena had departed sometime the week before while I was off duty— we never saw her again. Lilly's room was soon occupied by a lovely boy I'm calling Mickey, a two-year-old child with a severe case of cerebral palsy. His parents had enrolled him in one of Kurtzberg's clinical trials to see if cord blood could alleviate some of his profound neurological issues, and we'd bump into them regularly as Mickey's dad wheeled him through the halls in one of the red wagons.

We had new neighbors at the Alden Place apartments as well. The unit down the hall, vacant since Khaleda's family went home to bury her, was now occupied by the Ayers family from Florida. Their daughter Emily had just been diagnosed with leukemia less than a month before their arrival; shortly thereafter they'd learned her older sister, Kendall, was a perfect match. "It was eerie moving in," said Emily's mom, Stacy, knowing of the suffering that had just taken place in the quaint three-bedroom. "We just *have* to believe Emily is going to be healed, not just hope, but *believe* and have no doubt." As the Ayers walked through this whirlwind, they were treated to the traditional Alden Place housewarming—within a week of arrival they endured a home invasion and car theft.

The unit across from us now housed the Morrows from New Jersey—Susan, Keith, and their daughters, Eliana and Evelyn. Without exception, every stage of the Morrows' journey had been an order of magnitude more intense and harrowing than ours. It was as if their lives were being pumped through that *Spinal Tap* amplifier with volume knobs that went up to eleven. I was in awe that they'd kept it together.

Evelyn had been born with Hurler syndrome, an unspeakably heartbreaking condition that affects the organs, skeleton, and the eyes. When she first got the diagnosis, Susan couldn't resist googling it. "Then I slammed my computer keyboard down," she told me. "I said, 'There's no way God would do that to me.' Then I lay down on the couch and started crying. I didn't get up again for three days." At the first post-diagnosis doctor's visit, as she learned all the details of the disease in person, Susan vomited into a wastebasket.

A transplant would retard the progress of Evelyn's disease but never cure it. If they were fortunate, she'd make it to her midtwenties. Still, after hearing about life-extending results a cord blood transplant could deliver, Keith left his job as a bartender, rented a U-Haul, packed up his family, and headed to Durham, even before all the medical and housing arrangements had been locked down.

They'd set up a meeting with Dr. Prasad and his team in the Morreene Road office, but as they took their seats around the conference table, Prasad gave them bad news—their local doctor back home was insisting on performing the transplant herself. She refused to release the child to Duke. Without that release, insurance wouldn't cover the procedure.

"I pushed my Evelyn across the table at him like a hockey puck," Susan recalled. "Then I walked over to the window and pointed to the U-Haul. I said, 'That truck is us. We are here, and we are not going back. You need to fix my baby.' Then I heard sniffles around the room. Nobody was talking. After a few seconds, Prasad just said, 'You figure out the insurance; I'll take care of the patient.'"

After weeks of pleading—and threats—Susan finally persuaded the local doctor to release Evelyn to Duke. Eventually they moved into Alden Place. Evelyn had gone into transplant two weeks after Sebastian engrafted. Evie's dad, Keith, and I would eventually become buddies, but as usual our contact was severely hindered by the imperative to keep the kids safe. Meaning, apart.

Sebastian caught glimpses of these new faces after his numbers improved enough for Dr. Prasad to issue daily four-hour passes off the Unit. The number of infusion pumps on his pole was shrinking. The fentanyl went first, followed by the Actigall. This meant the chemo drugs were out of his system for good and his liver was no longer in danger of the dreaded VOD. With each day his orbit was expanding ever so slightly—from bed to room to hall to Unit to hospital to car to apartment. Every step out of the bespoke air of his tiny, HEPA-filtered room into the unmanaged atmosphere of Healthyworld qualified as a victory—to Sebastian's mind it was a matter of returning to safe and familiar places; for his brave new immune system it was Armstrong's moon walk.

Each time we returned to the Unit, the room felt smaller, the simple routines more tedious, the harder ones more torturous. The week after engraftment, Sebastian's NG tube fell out—a commonplace, nobiggie occurrence with zero net impact on the overall outcome of the transplant. It simply needed to be reinserted.

Here's the thing, though—the initial insertion occurs during surgery while the patient is under anesthesia having the central line placed; the procedure for *reinserting* a nasal tube that has fallen out is downright medieval. The nurse on duty, someone I hadn't met before, instructed me to sit on the bed, position Sebastian on my lap facing outward, put him in a headlock, and force him to sit still while she snaked the tube up through his nose and down his throat while he was fully conscious. "It will take less than a minute," she reassured me. "I've done this a thousand times."

The same thing had happened once before when Felicia was on duty. "The procedure was awful," she'd reported at the time, "but we got it done."

Not this time. The tube got jammed somewhere between his nose and throat, eliciting a high-pitched banshee wail of pain and terror. Sebastian's head twitched spasmodically between my hands, as if he were being electrocuted. I tried to comfort him as the nurse withdrew the tube, made some adjustment, and prepared to give it another go.

"*Nooooo!!!!*" he screamed. "*Daaddeeee. . . . !!!*"—I hadn't heard the word said with such panic since the plane ride down.

Enough. "Are you *sure* you know what you're doing?" I seethed at the nurse. "I know you just told me you've done this a thousand times, but *that* was a *total fail*."

I hadn't yelled or cursed, but my voice was dripping battery acid and my eyes matched Manson's mug shot. She scurried out of the room and I never saw her again, which is why I can't remember her name.

Minutes later Dr. Martin came in with another nurse to talk things through and, if necessary, call security. Desperate to avoid a replay of the botched tube insertion, I collected myself and appealed to reason. "Is the tube really necessary at this point? He's able to swallow now and he's been starting to eat food again. Can we forgo the tube on a trial basis at least?"

Martin consented, with a stern proviso that if the caloric intake dropped, the tube would be going in. When they left I went over the situation with Sebastian to make sure he understood the deal. He put down six pizza puffs that night. Given the ravages the chemo had inflicted on his taste buds, they probably tasted like cubes of plaster, but he understood this was preferable to the agonizing alternative.

The weekly dressing change was another regularly scheduled nightmare. The insertion point where the three lumens of the central line merged and entered his chest was the most vulnerable point on the surface of his body for infection. A small disk with a sterile cotton dressing and a large rectangle of adhesive tape always covered it, but they got grungy over time and had to be swapped out regularly. Doing so required two nurses in the room wearing masks, coats, and special sterile gloves to remove the large adhesive—a process as pleasant as a slow-motion chest wax. The pain left Sebastian in tears. And even after we'd done the drill several times with no surprises, it always rattled Felicia. "I could do this a hundred times," she said, "but I'll never make peace with the sight of a tube sticking out of my baby's chest."

Those moments weren't fun, but anyone who's spent time on a transplant unit would say they are just part of the cost of doing business, and relative to other patients, a mild cost at that. The point is not that every aspect of Sebastian's ordeal belongs in the *Guinness Book of World Records*. Just the opposite—like many of life's unpleasant, recurring phenomena, they followed a predictable trajectory—something at first shocking became a challenge to overcome, then a normal part of life, then an annoyance, then a banality. Dressing changes, tube problems, difficult bathing routines—after six weeks on the Unit, I regarded them the same way I'd come to regard the smell of urine on the street when I lived in the East Village. Off-putting but unavoidable nuisances.

And yet, despite all the solid reasons for wanting to leave, part of us wanted to stay. We'd not only acclimated to Hospitalworld, we'd mastered it. Felicia in particular had acquired the status of a seasoned pro. "I remember walking the hallway with her," said Susan Morrow. "She was the cool kid on the block."

As for myself, aside from that single flash of temper during the NG tube episode, I'd stayed true to my vow not to distress Sebastian with displays of anger or anxiety. I took great pride in a casual remark Dr. Page made on her rounds one day. "He does well when you're around," she said plainly. I'd never done anything remotely heroic in my life; my comportment on the Unit will always be the closest I come.

I'd hoped the rigors of transplant would straighten me out the way basic training does for many wayward young men who join the army to avoid jail. Sadly the Spartan discipline wasn't translating that well to Healthyworld. I was having crying jags behind closed doors at the office, sometimes triggered by bad news about another kid, sometimes by a random memory or photo of Sebastian as a baby. At home, shamefully, I started snapping at Lydia when she didn't pick up piano pieces I was trying to teach her on an electric keyboard I'd bought on Craigslist. More than once I reduced her to tears.

"I've read a few parenting books," Felicia reproached me. "None of them suggest yelling at a child or student until they cry. You have *got* to find a better way to encourage Lydia to play or she will shut down."

Felicia did a better job regulating her emotions on the outside, but she was experiencing some of the issues with memory and executive function Professor Cacioppo describes in her studies of solitary confinement. At the grocery store checkout, Felicia tried to pay with a credit card. The cashier asked her home zip code. It should have been a no-brainer—Larchmont, New York, is so proud of itself, local shops sell 10538 bumper stickers and coffee mugs. Plus, we lived there. Nevertheless, Felicia drew a complete blank.

In short, while the clean, sacred, caring, monastic environment of the Unit had brought out the best in us, it was entirely possible that the dirty, profane, harsh, distracting environment outside would bring out the worst.

This was the world, with its countless moral and microbial contaminants, into which we were soon to be ejected. And as we were about to learn, keeping our son safe meant taking over many of the crucial, delicate tasks the nurses had been handling so deftly. Discharge didn't mean discontinuation of treatment; it simply meant treatment would no longer be administered on an inpatient basis. The central line was staying in; the caregiver at home (mostly Felicia, sometimes me) would be responsible for administering intravenous and oral medications.

But wait, there's more: the caregiver was also expected to handle line care, flushing the lumens, changing the caps, checking for leaks. All of this had to be done in mask and gloves, with extreme caution and dexterity. Even a second's contact between a syringe and a random pant leg or arm could contaminate the line.

On a tropical mid-July morning, as Tray the music guy sang "Yellow Submarine" to Sebastian in his room, Felicia and I sat down on the Caregiver Room couch with a discharge nurse I'm calling Ingrid for an extended tutorial. She was a prim middle-aged woman with a hippie streak who presented as a librarian, one of the nice ones who'd cut you slack on late fees. Over the next two hours she walked through the steps of central line care with a tray of sample syringes, caps, and clamps to use for practice. "Each procedure has to be performed in a precise order," she instructed as she handed us a six-page laminated teaching board, replete with instructions, diagrams, and warnings. They went on and on. "The antiseptic wipe has to be applied for fifteen seconds minimum—you should count out loud—to guarantee adequate sterility. When you wash your hands, make sure you use a clean paper towel, both to dry your hands and to turn off the faucet."

"Can't we just use the Purell?" I asked.

"Yes, you can use Purell, but don't use it more than five times in a row before washing with soap and water. After that, it becomes ineffective." Who knew?

The instructions continued. Ingrid demonstrated how to do a blood draw using red food coloring. Then she walked through the directions for flushing the catheter, emphasizing the vital necessity of memorizing the SASH method: saline, application of medication, saline again, heparin, each injected with its own syringe. Sterilization of the cap was required before and between each step. Failure to perform these procedures properly could result in line contamination and infection.

The grass on the lawn outside had grown half an inch by the time she finished. "Any questions?"

"Yes," said Felicia meekly. "How am I suddenly competent to perform sophisticated work that people go to nursing school for?"

She was hyperventilating. Mastering these intricate techniques would be a challenge for anybody; for those who've just gone through the most frazzling experience of their lives, it was like being asked to create a Tibetan sand mandala right after going three rounds in an MMA Octagon. And given the potentially disastrous consequences from a single, minor mistake, it was no wonder Felicia felt overwhelmed. This was the first time I'd seen her so unnerved. "I was paralyzed with fear," she told me later.

We'd worked through a classic approach-avoidance conflict getting to this hospital in the first place; now we were working through a symmetrical one trying to leave it. Felicia recalled, "My sense of dread about the prospect of being discharged was creeping up. I know that sounds weird, but the Unit was such a safe place. It was so daunting to leave."

Hungry for guidance, she reached out to a former CGD mom who had shepherded two boys through transplant at once, handling posttransplant meds and line care on her own. After Felicia expressed doubts about her own capabilities, the reply was kind but curt: "You *can* do it; and you *will* do it."

Thankfully, the support system, which had sprung up almost spontaneously around us, was keeping us sane and on mission. It included the professionals at Duke; old friends like Tina Merrill and Jessica Yang, who volunteered to help with Lydia or household duties; new friends like Hunter Glass, who let me come down to the firing range on his property and blow off steam with a collection of firearms big enough to impress the Branch Davidians; other parents from Lydia's school who'd organized to prepare and deliver meals to the apartment; coworkers at the local affiliate who'd embraced me as one of their own; and of course all the friends and family who'd donated to our COTA fund. Many of them were classmates from high school or college I'd lost touch with—they weren't even Facebook friends, they'd never met Sebastian—and yet, in a world abundant with needier cases, they'd carved out time and dollars to help. Felicia defined God's grace as the granting of a divine gift one doesn't deserve. We received it in abundance.

Some friends made the effort to visit in person. A few were buddies of mine who figured, correctly, that I could benefit from some male companionship. During those weekend adventures we'd hit the bars and nightclubs of downtown Durham, a revivified urban district trying so hard to be the next Brooklyn, it had its own artisanal ramen shop. I was partial to the DJs at a spot called the Pinhook, and while the world has no need of middle-aged men trying to dance in public to old-school hip-hop, I supplied the spectacle nonetheless.

My parents also swung through at various points during our stay, which was no easy feat. My dad's body was breaking down in a variety of ways and walking had become a challenge. Yet as he aged, he'd morphed from a domineering family patriarch into a Ghost of Christmas Present, perpetually jovial and blithe. He was an upper. My mom had just recovered from her cancer surgery and was on her own taxing chemo regimen. Nevertheless, she flew to Durham and came on the Unit to relieve me and Felicia. Unlike my dad's happy-go-lucky attitude, her presence was an anchor of stark rationality. Both were valuable; I was grateful they came. Separately.

Most touchingly, our nanny, Mercedes, came from New York for a full week. She'd been with us since Lydia was born and throughout

those grueling years of Sebastian's diagnostic odyssey and toddler-
hood. Sebastian leapt with joy as she walked into his room, impervious to the shocking surroundings. *"Ay, cariño, dame un besito!"* She
figured out the hygiene routines in an instant and proceeded to play
with him for hours.

All nanny relationships are complicated; they start as employees,
they grow into family members, then one day they vanish. But as Mercedes held our son and spooned Kraft Mac & Cheese into his recovering mouth—*"Solamente un poquito, mi amor"*—it was as if he were six
months old again, tasting mashed carrots for the first time, his bed a
high chair, the hospital room a nursery. Her time with him was limited; her love for him was infinite.

Hang around doctors long enough, you learn to detect messages in
their body language and tone of voice. These are often more direct
than their words, which can sound like they've been written and jury
tested by a malpractice defense lawyer. As Dr. Prasad and the team
made rounds throughout July, an air of confident nonchalance replaced the silent tension and manufactured positivity that had defined
their demeanor weeks before. As the first chimerism test approached,
that nonchalance said, *Yes, there are no guarantees in this business, but
we're not worried about this. You shouldn't be either.*

When the results came in, the only surprise was to the upside. "In a
chimerism test, a count of forty-eight percent donor cells is considered acceptable," Prasad explained. "Anything above seventy-two
percent is considered very good."

Sebastian's blood came back with more than 98 percent donor cells
(the testing has a margin of error of 2 percent, so you can never hit
100)—and, importantly, none of the original recipient cells were de-

tected. Complete chimerism, a Mickey Mantle upper-deck-hitting home run. As Prasad and the nurse practitioner explained the results, I understood why every transplant center we spoke to was so eager to have Sebastian as a patient, the contingencies of a four out of six donor match notwithstanding. Coming onto the Unit, he had the profile of a sure thing—young, healthy, no prior exposure to chemo, afflicted with a condition with a known curative treatment regimen. These places, after all, are in the business of curing kids and creating chimeras. In almost every regard, Sebastian was good for business.

What was this new organism? Who precisely was I looking at on the bed? It would defy reason to say this process hadn't changed Sebastian—the nurse practitioner was holding a piece of paper that showed, with molecular specificity, how he'd been altered biologically. And any child psychologist would state unequivocally that, no matter how much of this he'd consciously remember years from now, it would alter the trajectory of his development one way or another.

And yet, here was the same Sebastian we knew and loved, laughing and playing with his sister, cracking up at fart jokes (and actual farts), and making his characteristic caveman grunts when he didn't get his way. As his body emerged from the depths like that battle-scarred sub in *Das Boot*, his old personality was resurfacing with it, with one new quirk: reconstructed, postchemo taste buds gave him a serious sweet tooth. Devouring candy at every opportunity (and on the neutropenic diet, those opportunities abounded), he earned a new nickname that he carries to this day: Sugarboy.

It occurred to me that during our stay here I'd experienced an intimacy with my son I'd never had with any other human. I'd examined and touched every square inch of his body surface daily; I'd had more direct, uninterrupted interaction with him here than ever before. To keep him alive and happy, I'd paid intense, continuous attention to his every word and noise. We'd spent countless hours together doing next to nothing, but I'd come to realize that when you are with someone you love, your time is never wasted. In short, I'd earned the right to call myself his father.

Life was good, or at least good enough, and now it looked like it would continue for all of us for quite some time.

We rolled our snake eyes the next week.

The cough returned. It was mild at first, but throughout the first night it grew as incessant and disturbing as Poe's telltale heart. On July 16, Day 30, a chest X-ray generated some troubling radiological language: "Low lung volumes with central bronchovascular crowding." A panel for common viruses was negative, but a CT facial scan found increased mucosal thickening in the sinuses.

Prasad was not troubled in the least. "Most likely it's the mucositis working through his sinuses, dripping into his lungs, and triggering the cough. Okaayyy?" Still, he saw the terror in Felicia's eyes—the cough didn't concern him, but her mental state did—so he delayed Sebastian's release a few more days.

Felicia worked through her anxiety about her pending home care responsibilities by training on the SASH technique ritualistically in the room under the supervision of Nurse Liz, memorizing each step, forcing back the fear of contaminating the line.

Finally, there were no more excuses; Felicia had achieved a modest proficiency with the line and syringes; Sebastian was still coughing, but serious infection had been ruled out; and his new immune system was finding its footing. It was time to depart Hospitalworld. July 20, Day 34, our forty-eighth day on the Unit, would (hopefully) be Sebastian's last.

The amount of stuff we'd crammed into that room was astounding.

We spent days purging what we didn't want and transporting the rest back to the apartment.

In preparation for the parade, the nurses asked Sebastian what color confetti he'd like. His choice was so odd they asked him to repeat it: brown, black, orange, green, and red. Maybe he considered the day an amalgam of Thanksgiving, Halloween, and Christmas. More likely he was just rattling off a list of colors to show that he knew the words. Regardless, they complied to a T.

Felicia's heart was pounding the entire morning. "Discharge day felt very much like my wedding day," she remembers. "You're starting a new life; you don't know if it's going to work out as you hope, but you're positive." A string of well-wishing staffers stopped into the room to congratulate Sebastian and say goodbye. Some brought presents. Others prayed.

Then it happened. Cradled in his mother's arms, dressed in a tie-dyed T-shirt he'd made in the Connection Room with his sister, Sebastian was disconnected from his pole for the last time and, face mask securely in place, he bade adieu to room 5214. The nurses cheered as they tossed the confetti—this moment and others like it would sustain them when the next tragic outcome drove them into the supply closet to weep.

Patients strong enough to stand came to their doors, their parents beside them. Some were new arrivals we'd barely met. Yet they ventured into the hall to bear witness and share the moment. As they made eye contact with Sebastian, a look of true solidarity passed between them—they knew what he'd just overcome; he knew they were staying behind. No one knew if they'd ever meet again.

Mercedes snapped a shot of the lucky patient surrounded by his beaming nurses; Lydia giving a double thumbs-up, Felicia smiling through tears. Then the door to the antechamber opened; my family removed its last pairs of paper booties and made its way to our packed, sterilized Subaru. Ingrid, the discharge nurse, came down to the parking lot and waved to Sebastian like a loved one bidding bon voyage from the Liverpool piers.

We'd see some of those nurses again, but many would fall out of touch, turning the page on our case and devoting their attention to the next kid who needed it. "That's my way of staying focused," one of them told me. "If I don't see them again, I know they are okay. That's enough for me."

Sebastian arrived back at the apartment sporting a mask, hat, gloves, and his dangling central line—the transplant poster boy. Our new neighbors were out, and though Sebastian did little more than wave as we arrived, Stacy Ayers later said that just seeing him gave her a big boost—the boy was her first living proof that kids who go into the Unit come out. "You guys did it," she recalled, "you'd made it that far. It gave us hope. We looked up to you."

That night at the apartment Felicia administered the first scheduled intravenous medication, the daily dose of CellCept. Her adviser was correct: she could do it; she did do it.

Chapter 16

Repair

....

"DON'T TOUCH THAT DOORKNOB!"

I was going to the bathroom; my wife was reminding me how.

"Wha . . . ? Oh, right. Sorry. Forgot."

"We have to use a paper towel or wear gloves *every time*. And, remember—same thing for the toilet handle and the faucet."

We'd moved back into the apartment the day before and, fastidiously observing the post-transplant guidelines, converted the apartment into a less cramped and sequestered version of room 5214. Sebastian was barely past boy-in-the-bubble phase, so our extreme germophobia—the most intense in the four years since the diagnosis—wasn't an irrational phobia at all, it was doctors' orders. No shoes, no guests, no nondisposable utensils or cups. Separate bathroom and laundry service for the patient, who slept in the master bedroom with his mother while Dad took the guest room and Lydia had the two beds in the kids' room to herself. And, above all, the abovementioned disinfecting procedures for doorknobs, handles, and faucets—any commonly touched surface could transmit disease.

It would be like this for at least another nine weeks, till Day 100, the date of the next crucial chimerism test. If the results came back as hoped, and Sebastian was otherwise healthy, he could be cleared to return home. In the meantime, we just had to HODL.

We converted the dining area into a combination supply room and infusion center. Boxes of medicines, syringes, gloves, and wipes arrived almost daily. The kitchen counter became an eclectic medley of bottles of oral meds and the various cups and droppers with which they were administered. The living room, of course, became one giant tangle of toy train tracks.

Felicia's infusion and line care technique progressed prodigiously. This was no small feat—another mom told us later she contaminated her son's line the first day out. Sebastian did his part too. He understood what was happening and helped out the best way he could—by sitting still. After several days of such sterling behavior, he made me promise to get him a dog once we returned home and Prasad gave the acquisition his imprimatur. I'd successfully denied similar requests for years—pets were a risk for CGD kids, and I'd relied on this fact to abort such conversations. This time resistance was futile.

Just like they had been on the Unit, the day's waking hours were dominated by the scheduled meds. Some infusions took hours and required the use of a portable timer-pump called the Curlin—a home-use version of the pumps that had previously adorned his pole. A relic of the late twentieth century, the Curlin looked like a close cousin of the TI-99 home computer or the early Motorola thick-as-a-brick cell phones. Its Culture Club—era design notwithstanding, the device was a game changer. "There used to be a time when no patient was discharged until they were off *all* IV meds and the central line was taken out—they had to be in the hospital for many months," said Dr. Prasad. "Now we want to allow them a normal life as much as possible." The Curlin—which made home infusion of IV meds possible—was the little engine of that progress. Felicia could get it up and running, place it in a preschooler-sized backpack, and, with the whole apparatus slung over his shoulders, Sebastian could easily slide off his chair and go off to play. With life hacks like this, the patient-self aspect of his identity was, glacially, ceding the stage back to the child-self.

Patienthood had become a sort of profession for him, with its attendant routines and metrics. Every morning, as the rest of the working world headed off to its jobs, either Felicia or I would dress Sebastian in his patient clothes, pack a patient bag, and commute with him to his patient "office" at the Valvano Day Hospital, where his workday typically involved a blood draw, additional infusions, and regular weigh-ins. (I saw the bills for these visits—they ranged from three to six thousand dollars each.) While there, he'd often run into some of his colleagues, seated or prone in their own examination room work spaces—other kids from the Unit who'd been discharged around the same time he had; Lilly, Clara. If his blood aced its performance review he'd get a bonus of Fruit Gems and gummies from the candy section of the hospital gift shop and a wagon ride through nearby Duke Gardens, the beautiful campus and its Gothic chapel—a heavenly landscape built with the founder's tobacco billions.

The routinized nature of a commute eventually leads most professionals to ignore or resent it. Sebastian, gloriously, took profound pleasure in the trip to the hospital every time—not the patient's pride of incremental convalescence, but the child's pure bliss of sensory stimulus and wonder. Given the choice, he'd always want to drive on the "woods way" instead of the highway, snaking along the local roads through the soaring trees of the Duke forest. As the sunlight dappled the interior of the car, he'd open his window and, through his mask, inhale the fresh oxygen served up by acres of towering elms—no HEPA filter needed.

Approaching the hospital, just beyond the hundred-foot boundary of the no-smoking zone, we'd regularly exchange glances with the walking dead—the adult inpatients so hopelessly addicted to nicotine they'd carved out a little slice of Marlboro country on the border of the hospital grounds. Attired in their gowns and plastic wristbands, most attached to IV poles, some in wheelchairs, they formed a ghastly welcoming committee, hoisting Winstons and Luckys to their lips.

I'd witnessed up close the immense investment of resources that go into making a seriously sick person well, and it was hard not to shake my head in scorn as I drove past. "You'd better not end up like *that*," I warned my son, hoping that years from now he'd remember all that had been done to salvage the temple of his body and treat it with proper respect.

After we arrived at the hospital parking deck, he'd hop into one of the wheelchairs by the elevator and squirm with anticipation at the free ride he was about to get through the subterranean passageway under the street and into the hospital. This was his idea of fun.

One afternoon on the way home, his mind ventured into the future. "Mommy," he asked, "do you think when I get better, I can go to school?"

"Yes, you will," she replied, turning to catch the faraway look in his eyes. "You'll start kindergarten next year."

"I will have no . . . nothing," he continued, pointing at the lumens of his central line. "I will have no fevers, no throw-ups, no nothing." He wasn't asking, he was telling. His flimsy tenure on health be damned, he'd locked in on this goal. Either through normal child development, the crucible of the Unit, or some penumbral personality shift caused by the donor cells swimming around his chimeric body, he was changing—from object to subject, from the done by to the doer, from patient to person.

His universe expanded every week. We were still forbidden to go anywhere even moderately crowded—Sebastian learned the phrase "I'm not allowed" and began to deploy it against any proposed activity he wasn't inclined to do—but he was allowed out as long as he stayed at least six feet apart from any stranger. Large, sparsely populated public spaces became favorite hangouts: the nearby Target on a weekday afternoon; the Duke art museum before the school year began. The cloth surgical masks he wore everywhere were a big help—Dr. Martin told us these masks, contrary to popular belief, do quite little medically to shield the wearer against airborne pathogens, but they work wonders *socially* by scaring potentially infectious people away. The net benefit of wearing one is quite real. Wherever we went, the locals, accustomed to the presence of transplant patients, cheerily helped while respectfully keeping their distance. They knew the drill as well as his nurses.

Sometimes we'd never get out of the car and just spend the whole day driving around. Sebastian was still forbidden to eat fresh fruits and vegetables, but fast food was on the approved list, so we'd make frequent trips to Bojangles', his beloved fried chicken drive-through. Then we'd trek out to the Durham rail yard to bask in the raw power of a Norfolk Southern freight train plowing through. Train traffic was sparse, so while we waited, Sebastian would get out of the car and walk among the parked diesel locomotives and graffitied freight cars, climbing over little hills of creosote-treated ties and plates. Heaven.

One wouldn't necessarily consider outdoor competitive sports a smart way to avoid germs and viruses, but there is one game where players typically stay far enough apart not to transmit disease—golf. The Hillandale Golf Course, just a few miles from the hospital, had a program to provide post-transplant kids complimentary equipment and access to the course. There was a dedicated golf cart for the kids, the world's most frequently disinfected six-seater, in which we could cruise around at our leisure. We had to be mindful of the amount of time Sebastian spent in the sun, but even in the Jonestown hotbox that was Durham in August, he insisted we hit the links a couple times a week, make like the Dukes of Hazzard in the cart, and occasionally even do some putting. His ubiquitous newsboy hat, though not a tam-o'-shanter per se, reminded the regulars of Payne Stewart, and he soon became a minor celebrity around the clubhouse. These were among our first experiences since the initial diagnosis where we could be outdoors without fear of grass, dirt, and sand traps. If the chimerism test was to be believed, the old CGD cells were gone forever.

When he regained sufficient strength and stamina, we bought him a little red bike with training wheels. He took to it instantly, and soon we were adventuring onto the American Tobacco Trail, a twenty-two-mile rails-to-trails project that has become Durham's most beloved biking/jogging path. I'd re-resolved to get in shape, and I'd run along or behind him, recalling the recent days when his favorite exercise was doing laps on the Unit on the storage room trike. Now within a month of discharge he could go for three miles pedaling by himself outdoors, the lumens of his central line dangling below the crossbar. The news merited an eyebrow raise from Prasad when we told him. "I was pleasantly surprised," he remembered. "Sebastian had a number of issues pre-transplant, especially in the lungs and in the gut. Given that, I was worried that his post-transplant course could have been quite difficult. He was doing better than we expected."

Sebastian's body was changing noticeably, sometimes overnight. He'd relearned how to chew and swallow and was ready to expand his culinary taste beyond sweets, though the Sugarboy moniker still applied. As more protein went down his throat, much of it Bojangles' chicken, his muscle mass returned. Like many post-transplant patients, he was also on a low-dose steroid, which added bulk. Put an extra three pounds on an adult and you can barely notice; put it on a thirty-pound kid and he's grown 10 percent. Day by day he was climbing his way back up the body-mass bell curve.

Then there was the hair. After months of gradual thinning his mop top was long gone; now he resembled a miniature middle-aged insurance salesman from league night at the local bowling alley. The nurses gladly shaved him clean. When I saw his bald head for the first time I recalled one of the first things a nurse ever said about him—back in the delivery room, when someone complimented the perfect symmetry of his dome like a tourist beholding the cathedral of Florence. Sebastian was proud enough of his own cranium not to complain about his new look.

Just as hair vanished from his head, it sprouted up everywhere else. One of the guaranteed side effects of the antirejection drug cyclosporine is the sudden profusion of dark, thick body hair. In a flash— think the transformation scene from *An American Werewolf in London* —his eyebrows turned black, doubled in width, then merged. He grew a Frida Kahlo mustache faster than you could draw one on his upper lip with a Sharpie. And it didn't stop there. His forehead, his cheeks, his spine were all soon covered in a layer of wispy black peach fuzz. I wondered if his donor cells might have come from a howler monkey and had a few vivid nightmares about him turning into a circus freak.

"Now's when you tell me this is going to go away," I implored the nurse practitioner during one of our daily clinic visits.

"Yes, no question—the hair will disappear as soon as we dial back the dosage. Plus, he's a boy; it's much easier on them than the girls." As always, it helped to think about those who had it tougher. Sebastian looked freaky but he was too young to care. For the teenage girls, a shaved head and mustache could not have been good for the self-esteem.

For Felicia the countdown to Day 100 may have originally felt like a burden, and as I observed her dedicating her entire life to caregiving, I reflected on how much this had cost her. When Sebastian was born, she was a thriving professional PR consultant with a growing business and a vibrant social life. This was not what she'd hoped to be doing at age forty-two, the peak of her productivity.

I never heard her complain. Instead she came to see the time in the apartment as a once-in-a-lifetime opportunity. The doctor-ordered sequestration meant we had family dinner together almost every night; we got into completing thousand-piece puzzles together on the apartment floor (Thomas and his friends relinquished some precious real estate). Family TV time became another sacred ritual—*MasterChef, When Calls the Heart, Jeopardy!*

"I see these months of nonstop quality time as a gift," she said one day in the car. "We've never appreciated the feeling of being in our own space, in a nonmedical environment, with him for this long. It's so precious."

She threw herself into kid-friendly activities at home. Sebastian had always loved baking (*MasterChef* was his show), so she started digging up all the recipes she'd wanted to try, often recalling things from her own childhood. Her masterpiece was a batch of cupcake cones—a dessert that looks like an ice cream cone but is really cake and frosting.

"This is a chance to create a joyous time for him. It's a shame every child can't have it."

"How is it any different from what other stay-at-home moms do, what you were doing back in New York?" I couldn't help needling.

"It's not the same—there's always the house to deal with, phones ringing, errands to run. It's really rare to have hours and hours to just be together."

As she was embracing this new routine, I spent my time doing what I was supposed to—working, providing, parenting. I was constantly worried that I'd mess up with the doorknob rule or some other procedure, get Sebastian sick somehow, and wind up back on the Unit. But aside from my odd habits of refusing handshakes and obsessively Clorox wiping everything I touched, to a casual observer I looked normal.

Internally, I was holding it together by adhering at least partially to my Program. I was exercising, drinking moderately if at all, staying on my meds, and meditating semi-regularly.

During our time on the Unit, the practice of loving-kindness had come naturally. It's hard *not* to feel intense compassion for the patients, families, and staff. Now on the outside, I took up my former practice of directing loving-kindness at strangers and noticed the onset of a new, peculiar psychological tic—the feeling of *metta* intermingling with unprovoked and quite inappropriate paternal impulses.

I took Lydia to see *Pete's Dragon* at the nearby movie plex; while buying popcorn I fixated on the flaxen forearm hair of the teenage concessionaire and for a moment I wanted to spoon yogurt into his mouth. The following week, as I filled up the Subaru at the Exxon Family Mart, I stopped inside to score a bag of Jack Link's teriyaki beef jerky. At the counter I locked eyes with a middle-aged Bengali clerk and imagined what it would be like to change his underpants. By the Alden Place pool, my gaze settled on an overtanned housewife sipping a Diet Pepsi. Her skin looked like brown luggage, and whoever had enhanced her breasts had defied the laws of physics, the laws of supply and demand, and quite possibly the laws of North Carolina. As she swallowed the soda I focused on the contraction of her face and throat muscles and imagined rinsing her mouth with the Toothettes and sodium bicarbonate solution we'd left by the sink back in room 5214.

Clearly the hard-core caregiving of Sebastian had built up its own forward momentum, warping my practice of loving-kindness. I'd grown inclined to relate to anyone I saw as a young person fighting for life. My father-self had become the dominant aspect of my identity, the lens through which I viewed all human interaction.

The husband-self, conversely, had atrophied alarmingly. During the months Sebastian was on 5200, Felicia and I hadn't even cohabitated. One of us had to be with him at all times, the other taking care of Lydia. We'd done the tag team thing admirably and avoided major blowups, but we simply hadn't been in the same physical space much at all. We were sharing the most intense, intimate experience of our lives, but separately—it was like a date where we watched the same movie at different showtimes.

Now, though we were having family time in abundance, we still weren't having much couples time. It speaks volumes that neither of us can remember what we did for our anniversary that year. For us, August 27 was simply Day 72, and the cause for celebration wasn't eleven years of continuous marriage but the triumph of Sebastian successfully coming off the CellCept and completing his final daily dose of the G. It was hard to recall that once upon a time we had a relationship that wasn't mediated through the nexus of a sick child.

Under the immense burden of childcare, we'd forgotten how to care for each other. It wasn't just that we didn't make time for each other, we literally forgot many details of each other's personalities and preferences. We would have bombed on *The Newlywed Game*. And some of our core personality differences, which had been complimentary in happier times, had twisted into abject antagonisms. Felicia's PR background made it easy for her to spin things positively; I had the journalist's tendency to see the skull beneath the skin. And—please pardon the stereotypes—her Scandinavian heritage reinforced the suppression of emotion, while my Latino roots fed off its public exhibition.

And the religion thing was still an issue. Since that moment by Sebastian's bed on transplant day, I'd been willing to admit that my humility before the power of the unknown had a spiritual component, but I still bristled at Felicia's overt Christianity. She'd crammed a semester's worth of divinity school curricula into our months in North Carolina—everything from C. S. Lewis to Billy Graham. Now she'd taken the lead in our intellectual arms race, which ratcheted up the tension inside the apartment.

"Are you aware," she inquired one night at dinner, a plastic forkful of pasta in her hand, "of the various books and studies confirming the power of prayer?"

"I don't dispute the power of prayer, I just think it helps the pray-*er*, not the pray-*ee*."

"So you acknowledge that it could help you, but you still won't do it. Didn't you have the same misguided resistance to antidepressants?"

"That was a scientific solution to an emotional problem, not an emotional solution to a scientific problem."

"You talk about science as if it has all the answers. You know many things happen on the Unit that the doctors don't understand?"

"They don't understand them *yet*. That's why they're practicing science, so they can understand in the *future*."

"You assume we have infinite potential to understand the material world. But quantum physicists will tell you matter behaves pretty strangely when you look closely enough." (That week, Freeman Dyson had been sharing space on her nightstand with Saint Paul.) "If the universe can accommodate the mysteries of the quark, can't it accommodate the mysteries of faith?"

When these conversations didn't degenerate into some *ad hominem* attack, they ended in another tacit acknowledgment that we were in starkly different places as people. It was likely that if we stayed together, we'd spend the rest of our lives tuning each other out and living like roommates.

One of the Duke social workers, who'd stressed the importance of a consistently calm home environment for Sebastian's healing, had provided a list of local marriage counselors. Now that Sebastian was past his toughest stretch, Felicia felt we had the time and bandwidth to turn some attention to our relationship and get the help we'd resolved to get just before the health crisis back in March had hurried us down to Duke. This was the one part of the Program I'd neglected.

The following week, a trivial disagreement about who would accompany Lydia to a Durham Bulls baseball game with Tina blossomed into our first full-blown fight. I erupted like Krakatoa. Felicia didn't talk to me for days.

As Hunter Glass once said, "Play stupid games, win stupid prizes." We knew it was time to make the call.

"My client is your relationship," said our new therapist, Robert Ferguson, PhD. His office, just past the Sam's Club a mile down the road from our apartment, occupied one of the suites on the ground floor of a modest mixed-use office building, the type that houses so many of Durham's small businesses. It was a long way from the Park Avenue office where Dr. Moore had written me my first prescriptions. Ferguson, a former actor, had switched careers and made a specialty of conflict resolution for couples. "Our culture doesn't put an emphasis on how to resolve conflict with people you're really close to," he explained. "You either learn it from watching your parents, or you don't. But love involves *some* conflict inevitably. You can't be close to somebody without discovering differences and hurting each other's feelings sometimes."

By the time we began our sessions, Lydia had started third grade back at Carolina Friends School. We had intermittent home care for Sebastian, so sometimes we brought him to our sessions, parked him in a cushy chair, and encouraged him to color or play on an iPad while Mommy and Daddy vomited all our crap onto Ferguson's couch. Felicia, ever the master at explaining things in language he could understand, told him Mommy and Daddy were going to our "talking teacher." No, it wasn't ideal. Yes, it was strange. What are you gonna do. . . .

In the first session we provided the obligatory recap of our relationship and medical odyssey. By the time we left, Ferguson had concluded the marriage was deeply dysfunctional.

Later, after taking a family history, he decided our childhoods hadn't prepared either of us well for adult intimacy or adult conflict. "Did you two once have the proper skills for managing conflict and lose them because of all this stress?" he wondered. "Or did you never have them at all?"

We had one thing going for us—an asset that has proved invaluable over the years—naked honesty. After being split open and turned inside out by our experience with Sebastian, we felt no need to deny or rationalize what was wrong with us. We were messed up and we didn't give a fuck who knew it because, frankly, we didn't have any more fucks to give.

"Your directness gives me a feeling of measured optimism," said Ferguson.

Time was limited—with luck we'd be heading back to New York before we could even complete ten sessions—so Ferguson went straight to hands-on problem-solving, coming at the relationship like an engineer trying to fix a broken machine.

Part of his method was assigning homework, starting with the book *The New Rules of Marriage* by Terrence Real. If your marriage is on solid footing, much of the text reads like it was ripped from *The Onion*; on the other hand, if your marriage is headed for the ICU, the book is both an eye-opener and a merciless mirror. It was here, and through Ferguson's frankness, that I became familiar with the concept of "grandiosity," and Felicia with "offending from the victim position," both of which we, respectively, needed to reckon with.

Using the book as a springboard for our sessions, Ferguson proceeded to prescribe a series of concrete, actionable tools for working through conflict. They are so simple and obvious it's embarrassing to admit we needed to pay to have someone teach them to us, but that was indeed the case. For those who might find them useful, here are the basics:

- When you've decided to do something—a family trip to the zoo, a couple's night out—don't forget that the top priority is having quality time together, not winning an argument about whatever might come up during that time. Getting along is often more important than being right. Avoid derailment at all costs.

- Designate a mutually agreed-upon time to discuss combustible subjects. Don't just engage spontaneously at the moment of peak annoyance.

- During those discussions, frame the issues in nonprovocative language. Avoid the "you" statements ("You're so X; You're just an X") in favor of descriptions of your feelings ("When you do X; it makes me feel Y").

- Try to guide such discussions to something you can call agreement or resolution ("Going forward, let's make sure we don't X so we can avoid Y").

- When this system breaks down and you end up in a fight, have some shared technique for ending it; learn how to shift into a repair phase.

I will confess to taking a semi-cynical approach to the entire endeavor. I'd come to suspect all couples' therapists of subconsciously craving the "rescuer" role in the famous Karpman drama triangle, addicted to the drug of rendering aid, with Felicia and me in the other two vertices: victim and villain, respectively.

My first instinct was to connive. The trick, as I perceived it, was co-opting Ferguson to the point where he'd conclude that in fact I was the victim and Felicia the villain, that it was *I* who needed to be rescued from *her*. Expressions of contrition and humility would lay the groundwork, and I figured that, like any teacher assigning homework, he'd be a sucker for an apt pupil. Rote memorization and regurgitation of key concepts and phrases would be the nectar with which I'd win him over. The strategy had certainly served me well in school.

For a while the rank Machiavellianism worked. I gradually started "winning" our sessions, which understandably drove Felicia nuts, which in turn made it even easier for me to win.

Then an odd thing happened—the therapy started working. We put Ferguson's rules into practice. At first, they made for semi-scripted exchanges in which we recited canned lines like this:

"Hey, sweetie?"

"Yes, honey." [Ferguson had also commanded us to use terms of endearment, even insincerely.]

"Do you have a minute to discuss something?"

"Sure." [Permission to air grievance requested and granted.]

"I've been cooking every meal for weeks. I have to say that, when *you* don't cook at all, it makes *me* feel like you think it's beneath you, and I feel underappreciated." [Complaint expressed in terms of feelings instead of direct accusations.]

"So . . . can we agree that I'll make dinner at least once a week?" [Complaint addressed with a resolution for going forward instead of denial or a pro forma apology.]

And yet, as absurd and contrived as the language of Ferguson's feedback cycle sounded at first, it was preferable by far both to silent resentment and to yelling, and over time we adapted the stilted phrases we'd been told to use into our natural speech patterns, attaining some modest fluency in the language of conflict resolution. You can indeed fake it till you make it.

In the midst of all this sensitivity training, the NFL season resumed in early September and I was glad for an excuse to play hooky from life and adjourn to the nearby Carolina Ale House for big-screen games, nachos, and bourbons. Conveniently located between the apartment and the marriage counselor's office across from the Sam's Club's Rhode Island–sized parking lot and between a Discount Tire and an Office Depot, the local sports bar was a great place to hang out alone, with Hunter Glass or with Keith Morrow, whose daughter Evelyn had just engrafted.

Keith, who mostly did night shifts on 5200, had recently attained the status of local hero. He'd been down in the hospital lobby when a wanted, wounded fugitive tried to admit himself to the ER. Hospital security alerted the police and a chase ensued. Keith sprang into action and tackled the perp. Since then the hospital staff had been treating him like Dwayne Johnson, but Keith said he was acting as much out of anger as altruism. "I had months of aggression built up," he told me. "I just blasted him."

We didn't discuss this episode at the Ale House. In fact, during our time together Keith and I talked about *anything* other than our kids' medical situations and the latest dispatches from Hospitalworld. That was the point.

As Day 100 approached it felt like we might actually pull this off and make it home safe with two sufficiently healthy kids and one sufficiently healthy marriage. Then on the morning of Day 90, the cough came back. Prasad suspected we'd be hearing again from Sebastian's lungs, and as usual he was correct. This was a high bronchial hack, the kind a child might make after accidentally getting some water down his windpipe.

It persisted for weeks. Prasad ordered a full workup—chest X-ray, pulmonary function test, you name it. The lungs were clear, but the cough wouldn't stop.

"This is the kind of cough that can make a mother feel like she's going insane," Felicia told me on the phone while I was away on business. "*Nothing* will end it." The diagnosis was a merry-go-round— at first the cough was caused by postnasal drip, then maybe asthma, then maybe seasonal allergies, then something serious enough to warrant a CT scan, then back to one of the first two guesses. The only partial fix was an aggressive anti-asthma treatment of nebulized albuterol and budesonide. This brought Sebastian's daily required medicines up to seven, and our average nightly hours of sleep down to five.

The nagging pulmonary problem raised an unsavory possibility— that the bad old cells had returned with a vengeance and reconquered Sebastian's immune system. Felicia also worried there might have been some disease hidden in the donor unit that slipped past the screening. To our immense relief and joy, Sebastian passed the Day 100 chimerism test with flying colors. Once again, his blood cells were greater than 98 percent donor, and the counts—white blood cells, hemoglobin, and platelets—were well beyond where the doctors expected them to be at that point. He was still coughing, centrally catheterized, and freakishly hairy, but on paper he was officially healthier than the day he first arrived.

Still, Prasad is famously conservative about letting patients leave Durham. He doesn't relish the power he has over these families' lives, but he doesn't relinquish it easily. "It's in the best interests of the child to be seen by somebody who understands their whole story and their post-transplant complications," he explained—a nice way of saying he doesn't fully trust many local hospitals. Nor does he trust all parents. "We have to seriously look at what housing the child has, what kind of hygiene there is in the home," he told me. "Sometimes we've had to find funds for housecleaning or replacing carpeting. That all happens at a discreet level."

Fortunately, he was confident in the team who'd be taking over Sebastian's care at Memorial Sloan Kettering back in New York, and satisfied that we'd keep our house tidy (Prasad has never seen our garage). But because of the cough, and his natural caution, he told us that the earliest we could return was late November—another two months. That hit with a thud.

Roll the montage. We passed October in our regular routine, though visits to Valvano scaled back to twice a week. Golf, Bojangles' chicken, trips to the rail yard, and bike riding filled the time. More thousand-piece puzzles—a Mercator map of the earth, Raphael's *School of Athens*. The new fall TV seasons—*This Is Us*, the presidential debates, and for reasons I can't quite grasp, the kids became rare fans of *Designated Survivor*.

The Ferguson sessions continued. I stuck with my Program. There were some notable setbacks—after the entire family forgot my birthday I blew my stack and called my own kids selfish assholes. Felicia slammed me in a Facebook post and started comparing me unfavorably to the Joker. But Ferguson got us back on track, focusing on personal responsibility, empathy, and repair, and encouraging us to make regular deposits in our emotional bank account.

One day in September I met up with Jon Seskevich, a nurse clinician at Duke specializing in stress and pain management education. By his tally, since 1987 he'd counseled forty thousand patient families, practitioners of faiths ranging from Islam to paganism. And as a student of Ram Dass, he was also an experienced meditator. We had much to discuss.

"Don't kid yourself," he said as we sat at a small circular table in the medical school cafeteria. "This post-transplant period is still a time of immense stress. It's all waiting and not knowing. The mind tends to go to the future—the what-ifs, the if-onlys."

"Mmmm. I feel like I could go on a meditation retreat for ten years straight and still never be able to detach from my feelings for my kids."

"I don't think detachment is the goal. The mindfulness is meant to create a field where sadness can be, anger can be. If you allow it to be without holding on to it, it can pass."

"Anger. Yes. The trouble is what happens *before* it passes."

"Sure, the easy-to-anger thing happens. It's like a cup—when it's filled with stress, you add anything else, the cup overflows. It's not that one thing, it's that the cup is filled. The meditation helps drain the cup."

"My wife would rather I pray. She resents the fact that I don't share her belief in the Lord's miracles."

"I don't share the beliefs of most of the people I work with. It's not about belief and convincing so much as finding a shared vocabulary, a way to acknowledge each other's feelings and experience. As for miracles? I've only seen one myself, but I've seen it thousands of times. The miracle is love."

On October 24, we wheeled Sebastian into the OR for another surgery—a good one, if there is such a thing. He'd been able to transfer his remaining daily meds to oral dosages and he no longer needed constant infusions, so the central line could now be replaced by a sub-cutaneous port, the size of a Kennedy half-dollar, to be positioned just under his right clavicle. There would still be a catheter in his chest for occasional IV meds, but he could finally ditch his Line Snuggler vest and be rid of the dangling lumens. No more strings for Pinocchio. A huge milestone.

Once again, we placed a fruit-flavored gas mask over his face; once again we watched the flight status monitor in the waiting room for signs of progress; once again we stood over our beautiful boy in the recovery room, waiting for him to wake up. The surgeon, who re-minded me of the Lieutenant on *The Wire*, told us he'd come to in twenty minutes. Then it was forty, then an hour.

Just wake up . . . just wake up. . . . You've almost made it. . . . Just wake up. . . .

When he opened his eyes, Felicia and I hugged and cried. We knew we'd be going home.

Part 3

Homecoming

November 2016–October 2018

Chapter 17

High on Gratitude

....

I was back in New York on business the night it happened, and I got the news from a colleague as I left the office. "We're going to call Pennsylvania for Trump. It's game over."

The presidential election of 2016 had been the most New York–centric of my lifetime, and as I walked through Times Square later that night to gauge the mood on the streets, it felt like September 12, 2001: stunned silence, muted despair, some overt sobbing. My Facebook and Twitter feeds were much the same. The flaming protests would commence the next day.

I, on the other hand, was ecstatic. Dr. Prasad had just cleared Sebastian to return home. His perma-cough had subsided, his blood counts and chimerism tests were rock-solid, and as an added measure Prasad had ordered a special neutrophil function test—the same one Dr. Herzog had ordered back when she made the initial diagnosis—to confirm the new cells were performing up to spec. It was official: my son would die someday, perhaps in a Trump-triggered thermonuclear war, but not of CGD.

As pedestrians around me and my friends online bemoaned the incipient apocalypse, I was giddy enough to make Gene Kelly look like Max von Sydow by comparison. Felicia and I were speechless when we heard the news. This was without question the best moment of our lives.

The election night divergence was a pronounced example of a distinct, emergent pattern. Our stay in Hospitalworld had remolded our mindset and our perspective, throwing us out of sync with Healthyworld culture. This friction first appeared when Tina Merrill, our dear friend in Durham, had graciously invited me and Lydia to a pool party at her lovely house a few weeks after Sebastian was discharged. I was eager to give Lydia some fun, normal experiences, so I'd accepted and made a yeoman's effort not to discuss our situation. I wanted to reacquaint myself with the art of small talk.

The grilled chicken was superb and Lydia had a blast with the other kids, doing cannonballs and playing Marco Polo; but somewhere between one guest's scabrous complaint about a resort botching a vacation reservation and another's lament about losing a bid on eBay, I knew it was time to leave. I couldn't yet engage with a world where these matters qualified as problems.

On the drive home, as Lydia sat in the back seat in a moist bathing suit and towel, we put on *Sgt. Pepper*. She sang Paul's parts and I did John. Near the end of "Fixing a Hole," my mind returned magnetically to the question at hand—How were we going to assimilate back into normal society? The sugar high of our recent good news notwithstanding, were we messed up in ways we didn't yet comprehend?

The Immune Deficiency Foundation lists "ongoing depression and anxiety post-crisis" as common emotional realities of a post-transplant family's "new normal." This wasn't that—not yet—it was just an unsettling, miasmic sense of *unbelonging*. Another CGD mom told me she felt the same way after her family returned from Duke. "We'd changed our lives so much to live in that other world, it was very hard to go back to normal," she said. "When you're at pre-K drop-off and other moms are complaining about diaper rash, it's hard to relate. And it's still hard to this day."

The election made it clear we were both emotionally misaligned with the rest of the world's stimulus-response reflexes. We simply didn't care who was president, and we couldn't join the millions of our countrymen who let the news of the day govern their emotional state, who approached politics as a religion. What was an outrage for many was for us little more than an image on a screen. In this regard, I'd achieved the meditator's detachment, and then some.

Conversely, we found ourselves increasingly sensitive to a ubiquitous aspect of pop culture the general public not only accepts but demands—on-screen violence. We realized this a few weeks before our scheduled return from Durham, when, on one of our rare prearranged, Ferguson-mandated date nights, we went to see the new Jason Bourne movie. The shooting and fight scenes were no gorier than the PG-13 rating warned, but we still found ourselves covering our eyes during the climactic hand-to-hand-combat sequence.

"I'm not sure I can take much more of this," I whispered to Felicia as Matt Damon and Vincent Cassel exchanged headbutts and choke holds in extreme close-up.

"Do you want to leave?"

"I would, but Ferguson told us to commit to having a good time. I don't think we should let minor things like this derail date night."

"So let's stay. It's almost over anyway. Just look at me." We spent the rest of the interminable scene locking eyes and kissing while Foleyed sounds of body blows and gurgling blood filled the theater in Dolby surround sound.

The unbelonging continued as our return to New York approached. Just as we'd been apprehensive about leaving the Unit for the apartment, we felt a festering fear about departing Durham and plunging back into a world that now felt so alien.

"I feel like we're leaving this warm cocoon," said Felicia.

But this was the whole point of the enterprise, tracing back to Sebastian's first mystery fever in June 2012—*get back on track*. Wasn't this what we'd always wanted?

In time, we reasoned, the entire Duke experience would recede into the past like a high school semester abroad—we'd retain some vivid details, but it would have little gravitational pull in our living present. So we set about the business of our return, and as usual the ineluctable concreteness of the logistics occupied mental space that would otherwise be commandeered by constant rumination. We packed, we arranged the reverse transfer of Lydia's schools. I had a hitch attached to the Subaru and reserved a U-Haul trailer for the drive home. *Deal with what's in front of you.*

The most delicate aspect of the move was of course Sebastian himself. Before Dr. Prasad released his patient, he wanted to kick the tires one last time—that meant one final battery of viral panels, chimerism tests, chest X-rays, blood counts, stool samples, thyroid hormone tests, and immunity status checks. Aside from a lingering vitamin D deficiency, there was no news. That was good news. By every measure, our son's new immune system was a masterpiece, as exquisitely designed, crafted, and finely tuned as an eighteenth-century Cremona violin.

The post-transplant protocol would continue after our return—until the one-year anniversary of his rebirthday, Sebastian still had to avoid most public places and social contact; he'd still need to wear a mask in public; and he'd still require semi-regular checkups and infusions through his subcutaneous port, administered at his post-transplant facility, Memorial Sloan Kettering. But until we came back to Durham for nine-month and twelve-month workups, November 23 would be our last scheduled meeting with Prasad.

The morning of the final appointment, Sebastian was confident as he sat on the exam room table, positive he was healthy enough to go home. Prasad was delayed by a crisis with another patient. At last he came, he saw . . . he concurred. "I recall it being a nice conversation," he later said with his inveterate understatement. "Felicia was teary. Sebastian was happy to get out of there."

I sized up the man who had saved my son's life, a man whose professional achievement and personal composure dwarfed mine. He'd done so much more than provide the service of an auto mechanic; he'd become a true role model.

"I'm trying to think of a way to thank you and the team," I sputtered. "What do families normally do?"

He jabbed the midair with his glasses as he replied jovially, "Just send a picture. Okaayyy?"

Felicia and I also had a final session with Ferguson. Over the course of our weekly appointments, he'd become more hopeful about our chances as a couple. "You weren't unique," he recalled. "I'd put you in a category of couples where I first think, Are they going to be able to change? Do they even love each other? Then, as the therapy progressed, the answer was, yeah, they can change because they've already changed. You'd become more open-minded. The love wasn't dead."

His parting gift to us was a set of commandments, handed down with Mosaic authority. They included the following:

1. **Principle: See each other as equals. No adult gets to control another adult, or is superior to or has rights to mistreat the other.**

2. **Principle: Protect the relationship bond during conflict by de-escalation of negativity.**

3. **Goal: Continually monitor and make deposits in the emotional bank account.**

4. **Goal: Prevent conflicts when possible.**

5. **Goal: Repair feelings and the relationship after a conflict.**

We wrote them down and vowed to keep them on Post-its on our re-
frigerator door back home. He told us unequivocally that wouldn't be
enough. His final, sternest commandment: continue therapy back
home. Otherwise, he assured us, we'd slide back into our bad habits,
especially if Sebastian's health became an issue. We nodded like doc-
ile children, but I was noncommittal. When does a shrink ever say a
patient has had enough therapy?

Ferguson was one of dozens of Durham friends and angels Felicia and
I invited to a going-away party we threw the weekend before Thanksgiving. In the spirit of the holiday we wanted to express our appreciation to everyone who'd supported us and say goodbye. Nurse Liz, Hunter,
Tina, Jessica, some parents from Lydia's school, some parishioners from
Felicia's church, some colleagues from my office—all assembled at a
local restaurant for us to express our gratitude. As Felicia and I labored
through some impromptu speeches, I scanned the room—it was odd to
have so many people from different compartments of our lives congre-
gated and comingling for the first time. But they shared a bond—the
rare generosity they'd shown us so freely. They'd also seen us at our most
naked and vulnerable. We'd only met them months before and we would
never see most of them again, but they knew us like few ever would.
"You'll find that as a man gets older, the most important thing is balance," Hunter advised me as we parted. "Like a good sleep-to-pee ratio."

On moving day Tina and her son, Sam, came to see us off from the
Alden Place apartments. We tried to thank her, but she was equally
grateful to us. "This was really wonderful for me," she said. "There's
nothing like the experience of being the best part of someone's shitti-
est day."

Our neighbors—the Ayerses and the Morrows—bid us adieu like
proud parents seeing kids off to college. We'd amassed a hoard of toys,
clothes, books, and boxes of new trains and tracks, not one of which
was to be left behind. After I crammed the electric piano and the red

bicycle into the U-Haul trailer, it was time. Tina snapped a photo of the four of us, haggard but happy. We hugged, strapped in, and drove off.

The drive home was memorable for what *didn't* happen. We *didn't* get rattled by the hideous traffic in the northern Virginia suburbs; I *didn't* lose it during the diabolically frustrating process of backing the trailer out of a driveway; we *didn't* freak out when a leak in the U-Haul's roof soaked half the boxes during a downpour that lasted the length of the New Jersey Turnpike. We were riding high on the ambrosial sweetness of our gratitude; a tidal wave of thankfulness that, we assumed, would carry us with uninterrupted love and equipoise into old age.

As we turned off the highway, Felicia began weeping. "I can't believe all the prayers have been answered," she said. "I know we still have a long road ahead, but we've completed the hardest part."

We took a deep breath before crossing the doorway back into our house. Everything looked the same, but it felt more like a soap opera set than a real home, with us as returning actors who'd stepped away from our roles for a season to appear in our first feature film. Presumably, everything was going to be different now. Better. The crushing pressure we'd always felt in this house was dissipating. Once Sebastian made it to his one-year anniversary on Day 365 we'd be in the clear forever.

I unloaded the U-Haul and, at the drop-off location, chuckled at a road rager who cursed me out for blocking a parking space. His "Fuack OWAFF!" was the first ripe, full-throated New York–accented profanity I'd heard in recent memory. We were truly home. I silently bestowed *metta*/loving-kindness upon him and headed to the house to enjoy our first night back in our own beds. Nothing was going to yuck my yum.

The unbelonging feeling kicked in the following morning when I dropped Lydia off at her old school. True to form, she traipsed into her new classroom and greeted her third-grade teacher for the first time as if she'd been there all year. Bloom where planted. Some of her old friends were there to welcome her back, and after reminding her to use the mini-bottle of Purell attached to her backpack zipper after every high five, I turned to leave and ran into some of the other neighborhood parents in the hallway.

They greeted me with long, forceful hugs—think Cicely Tyson at the end of *Sounder*. We hadn't publicly announced the exact day of our return, so the sight of us suddenly reappearing was a miraculous surprise. I sported a thousand-yard stare, overcome with bewilderment at snapping back into our old routine as if the past eight months had just been a fever dream. I accepted the hugs while suppressing the terror at catching something from one of their kids and made a polite but hasty exit.

This was the plan: over the next seven months, barring complication, the doctors at MSK would gradually wean Sebastian off his remaining medications. The CGD was gone, but the acquired immune system was still getting its footing. If all went well, we'd have his port removed at the twelve-month checkup back at Duke. Then he'd be free of his final medications and restrictions and, like Pinocchio, become a "real boy."

Another two hundred days of the immunocompromised lifestyle may sound like an eternity, but as much as we might have preferred this next phase to play like a scherzo movement, we appreciated the schedule's plodding andante. Honestly, we required our own weaning off of the mentality of transplant parents, a lifestyle dominated by meds and precautions. We had to approach this like deep-sea divers, ascending slowly to avoid the bends. The regular appointments at the post-transplant facility would not just keep Sebastian's recovery on track, they would ease our own transition. The pediatric wing of the Memorial Sloan Kettering Cancer Center would be our halfway house.

Our first visit was something of a homecoming—MSK is adjacent to the New York–Presbyterian Hospital complex on the East Side of Manhattan where we'd first taken Sebastian for his mystery fever in 2012, and where he'd originally been diagnosed by the immunologist Ronit Herzog. For all its worldwide renown MSK is not experienced in cord blood transplant for CGD patients, which is how we wound up at Duke, but it has managed the post-transplant care for thousands of kids.

The volume of business done on the MSK pediatric floor is evident the moment you check in and walk past the fish tank (decorated with lovely iridescent coral and stocked with blue dory). The waiting room is larger than the Mall of America food court. The ceilings are thirty feet high. There's a cell phone charging station with twenty ports. Desktop computers and resident tutors guide the kids in learning games while they wait. The recreation room is equipped with dozens of board games, vast supplies for arts and crafts, and a functioning oven for baking cupcakes. An armada of toy wagons lines the main walkway like limos on Oscar night; clowns make the rounds, juggling and making fart jokes. A rabbit warren of examination rooms extends ad infinitum behind the doors.

We found comfortable seats and waited—with a patient population that big, the likelihood of an on-time appointment is as slim as an on-time Friday night departure from LaGuardia. We scanned the room—aside from a noticeable demographic shift from Duke (fewer intubated torsos adorned with college basketball T-shirts, more little bald heads in yarmulkes), the expressions were the same. We recognized the ashen faces of parents freshly immiserated by a recent diagnosis—on one of our subsequent visits a despondent mother collapsed at the doorway of the phlebotomy room; the benumbed faces of moms who've acclimated to the ecosystem of Hospitalworld; and the chemo kids, calm and alert, trying to relax or amuse themselves while their tireless poles stood guard above them, infusion pumps transferring precious fluids from bag to bloodstream. We were back among our people.

It is a challenge to do kindness on such an industrial scale, but MSK pulled it off. The staff was not only caring and gentle, they were well informed about our case—we were spared the irksome "take it from the top." The primary doctor, Farid Boulad, was an Egyptian Jerry Garcia. Sebastian took to him right away, noting how his name rhymed deliciously with that of his Duke transplanter. "Boulad. Prasad. Boulad. Prasad," he repeated in a hip-hop cadence.

The MSK staff approached these appointments as pro forma checkups. Just a quick look under the hood, an infusion here or there when needed, a number to call in case of emergency. All matter-of-fact, no cause for worry. We appreciated the positivity, but we knew better. The post-homecoming phase is often a time of crushing setbacks. And just as we were acclimating to our old habitat, three other families from our time on the Unit were contending with awful news.

Lilly Hicks, the teenage leukemia patient who'd been Sebastian's next-door neighbor on the Unit, had returned home to Greensboro at the end of August. In November, she was hospitalized with extreme, prolonged fatigue. Tests revealed that her steroid regimen had induced a hyperglycemia similar to diabetes. For the next few months she had to go on insulin, adding daily injections and hospital visits to her already burdensome post-transplant drug regimen.

Emily Ayers, one of our Alden Place neighbors, went home to Florida just as Hurricane Matthew was hitting Cuba. As it approached Florida and the Weather Channel went into continuous coverage, she came down with cold symptoms and was having trouble breathing. Her oxygen saturation levels dropped to 60 percent. A CT scan revealed that her lungs were filled with fluid. She had what's called idiopathic pneumonia syndrome, which occurs in about 10 percent of post-transplant patients. If not treated properly, it can lead quickly to organ failure and death.

Emily wound up in the ICU at her local hospital. Her doctors gave her a massive dose of steroids, telling her mom, Stacy, there was only a 9 percent chance she'd live. Emily made it through, but "it was the worst time in our lives," Stacy told me. "Transplant was *so* much better."

The Morrows' story, as always, should be written in twenty-four-point boldface font. Their daughter Evelyn engrafted successfully, but her hemoglobin levels never recovered into the normal range. She was vomiting four times a day and required several ER visits and blood transfusions. The family made it home to New Jersey, but the episodes continued—"A week after we got back we almost lost her," her mother, Susan, recalls. "She was limp in my arms as we drove to the hospital." It would take five more transfusions before the hemoglobin levels normalized. In the meantime, Evelyn was also diagnosed with a treatable but incurable thyroid condition called Hashimoto's disease, which occurs in a small percentage of transplant kids.

As if that weren't enough drama, Evelyn was back under the care of the same doctor who'd originally refused to release her to Duke. The parent-doctor relationship had degenerated to a state of abject rancor, and Susan says it picked up right where it left off. "The first time I saw [that doctor] back home, I asked, 'Hey, are we cool?' She said no. So I just said, 'Okay, let's be cool not to be cool.'"

Those were the scary stories. At the other end of the spectrum, we heard a jaw-dropping survival tale that defied both the odds and the science. The same week we came home, ten-year-old Abby Furco was making national headlines. She'd been discharged months earlier from Duke after the doctors had declared her a lost cause. She'd spent weeks in the PICU and, shortly after marching in the Unit's Independence Day parade, headed home to Virginia for hospice care. She was given days, not weeks, to live. Yet November rolled around and there she was, on *Inside Edition*, in *People* magazine, and blowing up social media. Abby had come home, flatly declared she wasn't destined to die, and resolved to walk as a flower girl in a friend's wedding. Somehow, she made it down the aisle, beaming in a white dress and garland. Despite ongoing health issues she's still alive today, possibly the Unit's greatest superstar.

It's precisely those kinds of stories—tales of crushing setbacks, stories of miraculous survival—that can lead one to church. The post-transplant outcomes seemed so arbitrary, and we were now so far from the sanctuary of Duke, that it behooved us to stay on God's good side. We returned to our local Catholic parish for weekly Mass, though Sebastian was still under restriction, so he spent the first several weeks up in the choir loft in mask and gloves.

It was becoming clear that Felicia and I had narrowed the spiritual gap that had become such a fault line in our relationship. With the worst of the transplant over and removed from the dense Christian social milieu of North Carolina, Felicia dialed back the most heavy-handed aspects of her piety. After witnessing the strength and generosity of all the believers who'd helped us, the countless instances in which Christianity seemed to bring out the best in people, I was ready to dial up mine. Whether or not Jesus truly walked on water or rose from the dead was irrelevant—the power and the social utility of his words (at least the ones I could understand) was, to me, self-evident.

I scanned the pews during service, examining the faces of my fellow parishioners concentrated in prayer. These were not stupid sheep or wild-eyed zealots. They were other humans, grappling with their individual problems and sufferings, cognizant of society's countless ills, silently calling upon a divine force for the power and calm to face life's challenges and be better people. I doubted I would ever believe the way the devout did, but I was willing to fake it until I found out, to see if I could plug into that airport courtesy outlet of faith. Spend years parenting on the edge, and (to borrow a phrase from John Dominic Crossan) eventually you'll figure out what you stand for . . . and what you kneel for.

The primary pillar of our faith in those first months back was gratitude. Whenever any disruption or threat to our tranquility arose, we reminded ourselves how fortunate we were, how much we had to appreciate. In that spirit, I spent days composing handwritten thank-you notes to everyone who'd contributed to our COTA account. With each note I enclosed a wallet-sized photo I'd taken of a happy Sebastian during a visit to the North Carolina Transportation Museum weeks before our return. He's seen smiling and spreading his arms to embrace the world as he poses in front of a 1951 General Motors diesel locomotive.

The practice of writing 120 personalized notes is a deeply meditative and humbling exercise. I did an adequate job personalizing each message, but the tone never deviated from that of the caption I'd written to accompany the same photo when I posted it on Facebook:

> This moment of health and happiness was made possible by all
> of YOU—everyone who helped, prayed, donated, fundraised,
> accommodated, sympathized, paid insurance premiums, paid
> taxes, cooked, babysat, filled in, listened, wrote, visited,
> forgave, or did any of the other countless things—many seen,
> many others unseen—that have made Sebastian's survival a
> reality. Whatever other questionable behavior may trouble
> your conscience, you can assure yourself that you've helped
> save the life of a child who very much wanted and deserved to
> live . . . so you got that goin' for ya! Cheers!

As Christmas came around, we were flying high. Sebastian's recovery was progressing without impediment; our marriage was regrounded;

our spiritual life was both a rock and a buoy. Our lives were indeed back on track. We just had to get used to it.

Out of an abundance of caution we got a fake tree—with the kid still on antifungal prophylaxis we didn't want to risk *Aspergillus* infection from a decaying Douglas fir. That asterisk aside, it was the best Christmas ever. My parents came to celebrate with us, my mother driving up from Philly, my father and his second wife making the trek from Kansas City. Sebastian at the time had developed a strong taste for the "Linus and Lucy" song from Charlie Brown. He would bust out in uninhibited, spasmodic dance moves whenever we played it. On our living room floor, he and my dad—all 305 pounds of him—boogied to the Vince Guaraldi classic as the rest of us sat around the fireplace, looking on in contentment. This was our family's version of the "Jai Ho" dance from the *Slumdog Millionaire* credit sequence.

Make whatever moves feel right, I thought to myself. *Until the music stops, my son, the dance floor is yours.*

Within days the calendar would flip to a new year, and for the first time in a long time we were looking forward to it—new year, new blood, new hope, new life, new us.

Chapter 18

The Calving Glacier

....

For a while it worked.

Months passed without incident. I went to work, Lydia went to school, Felicia went about the business of caring for the house and the patient. Our home was a happy cacophony of morning television, piano practice, and the swarming motors of landscaping equipment. Sebastian spent most of his time playing at home with Thomas, riding his beloved red bicycle at a nearby playground, and begging me for a dog. He continued taking his meds and attending his regular post-transplant appointments, which grew less frequent as his new immune system steadied like a newborn foal learning to trot around the pasture. The only complication was a persistent rash in his armpits—a sign of mild GvHD that could be treated with prescription ointment. He also caught a few colds. When he spiked a fever we'd scoot down to MSK for a viral panel, but it was all cool—getting sick was now allowed. Compared to what other families were struggling with, we were golden.

On Day 270 Felicia flew with Sebastian back down to Duke for his nine-month checkup. He was still forbidden from the filthy confines of commercial airliners, so she arranged transportation with a wonderful organization called Angel Flight—a group of altruistic pilots who shuttle sick kids on their private planes. I stayed home with Lydia, tracking the progress of a little Piper PA-46 on FlightAware as it went through a patch of rough weather over Virginia. It was a pleasant change of pace to be preoccupied with aviation safety more than immunological vulnerability.

This was the first flight for Felicia and Sebastian since we'd made that awful trip down to Durham a year before. He had horrific memories of air travel and his anxiety was palpable. They had to wear headphones to dampen the roar of the engines, which, Felicia recalls, made him look even smaller and more helpless than he already did in his mask and gloves. "He tried to be brave, staring ahead with his clenched jaw," she reported later. "We held hands and said a silent prayer. Then the plane took off and there was just blue infinite sky all around. All our worries seemed so far behind us."

Sebastian aced the nine-month chimerism test and the rest of the diagnostics. Prasad directed the MSK team back in New York to begin weaning him off the cyclosporine. The freaky body hair soon disappeared. When he returned home, Sebastian no longer had to wear masks in public, but I kept a box of them in the Subaru's glove compartment anyway—they came in handy when I had to talk my way out of a traffic ticket.

As we'd promised, Felicia and I had written Ferguson's commandments on Post-its and stuck them to the fridge door. Like good disciples, we honored time-outs, adhered to the rules of the feedback cycle, and made regular deposits in the emotional bank account. All remained quiet on the home front.

Sebastian celebrated his fifth birthday modestly, as usual, but was so overjoyed at the occasion, he declared, "I'm in the five of life!" (As he grew and his vocabulary evolved, he was increasingly prone to *awwww*-inducing Hallmark Channel exclamations such as this.) Felicia latched on to the phrase and fashioned it into her own set of commandments, "The Five Fs for Life." Essentially a codification of her survival guide during transplant, they laid out like this:

1. Faith. With the belief in what is unseen and what is positive, anything is possible.

2. Family. Each family member has a crucial role to play. And together the family is healed and becomes stronger still.

3. Fun. Find ways to be glad and rejoice in every circumstance.

4. Fitness. Children are a mirror for our energy; taking care of ourselves ensures they're absorbing what is healthy and positive.

5. Friends. We will always be indebted to them, and we must honor their kindness by paying it back and paying it forward.

These also got their own Post-its and coveted space on the fridge.

We scheduled the one-year evaluation a few weeks before Day 365—if all checked out, Sebastian would have his subcutaneous port and chest catheter removed; no more surgeries, no more intravenous meds. This time we all went—Lydia with me on Delta, Felicia and Sebastian on another Angel Flight.

"You're looking great!" Prasad announced as he came in the examination room. As he drew a treble clef in the air with the arm of his glasses it took me a second to realize he was addressing me, not Sebastian. He and the nurse practitioner inquired about the nature of my Program, which I'd been upholding with mid-level discipline, as if there could be no other explanation for the uptick in my appearance and affect. "Having my son cured of a rare and lethal illness may have something to do with it," I answered, "but, yes, I've also cut back on carbs."

We'd reached the end of the road map—adios to the cyclosporine, the antibiotics, the antifungals. The surgery to remove the port, Sebastian's tenth time on an OR table, was a victory lap. For the rest of his life he'd sport a Frankenstein scar below his right clavicle and another, more clover shaped, closer to his heart—respective mementos of the port disk and the central line. For a child whose flesh had been cut and punctured as many times as his martyred namesake, Saint Sebastian, it was singular pleasure for him to know the curtain was finally coming down on the relentless, painful drama of needles and scalpels, the only existence he'd ever known.

Back in New York our good fortune continued with such consistency it no longer felt like fortune. Sebastian grew strong enough to partake in father-son roughhousing, and we began to entertain ourselves by performing some of our patented wrestling moves on the master bed—the Brooklyn Stomp, the Anaconda Death Squeeze, the Aztec Human Sacrifice. On Father's Day weekend, exactly one year after Sebastian's rebirthday, we went to the beach for the first time. He crossed his final frontier, a public swimming pool, the following week. Sand, dirt, rotten leaves, cut grass, and other snotty-nosed kids—all were stripped of their terrifying power. The world was one big welcome mat. The kid was fit to withstand the gaze, and germs, of millions.

I continued to believe that if he was okay, I'd automatically be okay too. Prasad's acknowledgment of my improved condition was a win, and I really knew I was in a good place when Hunter Glass told me he'd named his twelve-gauge pump-action tactical shotgun "the Miguel" in my honor. (The man makes a habit of christening his firearms.) He said the name fit because the gun "is dependable, it shoots straight, and it can fire a wide variety of ammunition, so the target never knows what's coming out of the barrel." With that endorsement, I was ready to take on the world.

My anxiety subsided dramatically—a monthly Klonopin prescription lasted half the year. And I was so pumped about our new lives I went cold turkey on the Wellbutrin too. I didn't feel depressed because my life was no longer depressing. Indeed, I had no excuse for feeling anything but joy and gratitude. And if Sebastian could stop taking his meds, why couldn't I? I still kept the pills in my briefcase—they'd shake in their plastic bottles like little maracas when I ran to catch the train—but that's where they stayed. Eventually I threw them out.

The folks from Make-A-Wish came by the house. I'd always thought the charity catered exclusively to the terminally ill or the chronically poor, but, no, Sebastian qualified despite his manifold privileges. As two fairy-godmotherly women sat on our little living room couch and asked what he had in mind, he told them he wanted to take a trip on a special train—western Canada's Rocky Mountaineer. Back on Unit 5200, Felicia had showed him pictures of its gleaming locomotive and glass-topped passenger cars coursing over turquoise rivers and through coniferous forests with snow-capped peaks in the background. If a week with Thomas on the isle of Sodor couldn't be arranged, this would certainly do.

It was then I committed to the idea of writing this book. With the kid cured, the marriage repaired, and my head becalmed, I envisioned its final scene—that train pulling out of Vancouver station, the four of us exchanging happy-ever-after smiles on its open-air observation platform as the lumbering diesel pulled us smoothly into a future of laughter and surprise, proudly basking in the knowledge that we'd made it. Cue the Zemeckis movie score. Our triumphant story could end . . . right about . . . here.

I noticed the first few hairs on Sebastian's pillow in June. Within a week, a large clump had fallen out halfway between his right ear and the crown of the skull. We had to comb it over, lest he look like the victim of a frat house prank. More came out with each brushing, and after every bath, a fresh exodus of brown hairs circled the drain. In a flash he returned to the middle-aged insurance salesman he'd become just before the nurses shaved his head the year before. WTF?

The team at MSK directed us to a dermatologist who saw a lot of post-transplant kids. She noted that his scalp was as flaky as pie crust; a common condition in babies called cradle cap that also pops up in transplant kids. "It's just a mild symptom of GvHD," she said. "The follicles aren't coming out. With proper treatment, the hair will grow back eventually." She sent us home with a bag of prescription shampoos and ointments. Not to worry. Felicia didn't give it a second thought—Lydia had had something similar as a baby. She knew it was nothing.

I went the other way. My rational mind listened and understood; but after three weeks of fixating on the kid's scalp, the rational mind was no longer in control—the Dragon was reawakened. As the forces of chaos reasserted themselves, whatever defenses my mental immune system could muster were no match. Anxiety punched through the walls of my mindfulness practice like plywood. At church, I troubled deaf heaven with my bootless cries. The Lord was silent.

By mid-July my mind was coming apart like a calving glacier. I took Sebastian to see Dr. Malech at the NIH. He tried to keep me calm but acknowledged there was reason for concern—in some post-transplant patients, alopecia turns up as a symptom of chronic GvHD, the kind that can wreak permanent havoc on organs. His advice was to stay on top of it and get back to him, especially if some other issue emerged, but his best guess was that it was just "an early misfunctioning of the new immune system. It will probably rattle around until things fall into place."

That did little to allay my symptoms—insomnia, loss of appetite and concentration, pacing. The thing about any visible health issue from the neck up is that you can't *help* but see it every time you look at the kid. My powers of perspective and denial collapsed. I could only envision worst-case scenarios.

I was weeping, spontaneously, uncontrollably, pathetically. We went to the *Lion King* for Lydia's birthday—Sebastian was in the habit of belting out the opening lyric *"Nants, ingonyama!"* while flinging himself onto the nearest mattress, so it felt like a good choice for his first Broadway show. I was chewing my fingernails bloody before the lights went down, and openly bawling by the second verse of "The Circle of Life." Tourists in the row in front of us turned around to take in the *real* drama.

I kept falling apart at family functions, on the way to work, at church. (The Lord's Prayer beseeches God to protect us from anxiety, for good reason.)

Why?

In part it was a profound disappointment that our run of luck was over—a reaction to the implosion of our perfect ending, the realization that Sebastian would never be completely normal. Sure, this was only a small setback, but what was next? His next checkup might reveal long-term damage from the chemo, a thyroid problem, some cognitive issue.

"You have to adopt the mindset of being in a state of remission more than being completely cured," said John Boyle of the Immune Deficiency Foundation. "The comparison to cancer might freak people out, but whenever there is transformative therapy like a BMT, you will have to stay on your toes for *decades* to come." We'd known as much ever since we'd signed each individual page of the treatment plan back at Duke, but it was no longer a mere paragraph on a consent form. It was reality.

I scampered back to my Park Avenue shrink—the one with the nasty Yelp reviews—to re-up my meds. With a sneer she chastised me for quitting the Wellbutrin without consulting her—a big no-no—and asked why I was such a wreck. When I explained the deal with Sebastian's hair, she proposed that I was projecting insecurity about my own advancing baldness.

Maybe, but that wasn't the whole story. As confirmed by other parents, post-transplant complications can trigger bouts of crippling PTSD, or at least garden-variety paranoia and neuroticism. Years of cumulative dendritic atrophy and amygdala swelling in a brain under chronic stress will do that, according to Dr. Amy Arnsten, the Yale neuroscientist and stress expert. Sadly, you don't just snap back to normal when the initial chronic stressor goes away.

Other parents were going through the same thing. In New Jersey, our former Alden Place neighbor Susan Morrow was melting down whenever she saw the shadow of feet approaching the closed door to her bedroom at night, even if it was only her husband, Keith, or one of their kids. "It reminded me of the nurses coming into our room on the Unit; I was constantly afraid people were coming in to tell me something bad was happening with Evelyn."

Down in Florida, the Ayers family kept little Emily in a bubble at home for a full year. "Even after we were cleared to start going out again, we started having issues not *wanting* to go out," says her mother, Stacy. "The first time she caught a cold I went crazy with the what-ifs. We're still like that. We see public spaces differently. You see normal; we see dirty." Emily's sister, Kendall, was using so much sanitizer she was burning her hands. Emily herself developed tics and started breathing strangely—at least her mother *thought* she did. "We took Emily to a psychologist," Stacy recalled. "He said, 'Your daughter's fine, ma'am, but we have to work on *you*.'"

Stacy says the germophobia is just part of the family's permanent lifestyle. "I felt like I missed the first diagnosis, so I'm compensating now. I got beat once, I'm not going to get beat again. So I worry about things that will never happen." As of this writing, Emily has yet to hug her grandparents.

Most parents understand this hypochondria by proxy has less to do with the kid's condition than their own. But over the next several months, whenever I stabilized enough to regain a grip, a new ailment would appear out of the blue to legitimize the worry. We made it to the Make-A-Wish trip, which the foundation arranged with precision and boundless generosity (I can't praise their work enough). During the first leg of the train ride I was able to suppress my anxiety over the hair issue with generous helpings of Klonopin and vodka. I kept myself in a semi-stupor as we rolled through the Canadian Rockies, my gaze bouncing back and forth from the scenery to my son's scalp.

For his part, Sebastian was living the dream. But after we rolled into Banff, he spiked a fever of 102. By Calgary, both kids were cooking. We got on the phone with MSK to see if we needed to come back immediately, and the Make-A-Wish travel department to see if that was even possible. Felicia tried to stay positive throughout the trip, but I felt so defeated I couldn't fake it. "It's hard to enjoy this trip to its full potential because a quarter of our group is gloomy and quiet and irritable, and clearly disturbed," she said as we swung by a pharmacy for more Tylenol. "Being with someone who is unable to experience joy infects the whole experience."

Felicia's mind was misfiring too. By her own account, she'd developed a troubling hypersensitivity. Certain sounds or smells would set her off, as would petty annoyances like water on the bathroom floor or my use of common phrases like "spike a fever" that, for some reason, got on her nerves. And there were nights she'd wake up in a panic, thinking she'd forgotten to give Sebastian his cyclosporine, even though he'd been off it for months.

By the time we made it home the scar tissue on our marriage was in a state of dehiscence. As Ferguson had predicted, discontinuing our counseling sessions virtually guaranteed we'd backslide. For months we'd been getting by on gratitude. It had bonded us together, but now it had lost its adhesive power. Like the high from a diluted opiate, the emotional fix we got every time we reflected upon our many blessings diminished over time. Sebastian's fresh health issues, however manageable, made it hard to be happy.

"With post-transplant setbacks, some people are just amazing folks, ready to strap the armor back on," said the IDF's John Boyle. "With others it's such a gut punch, it's very difficult. For some couples it may be the straw that breaks the camel's back.

"We advise couples to do four things: therapy, therapy, therapy, and therapy."

"I'm through."

Felicia was making her opening statement in the stuffy, document-strewn office of our new counselor, an LCSW named Kathleen Friend. The only reason Felicia had agreed to come this time was that we both felt it would be cruel to inflict the trauma of divorce upon our kids so soon after they'd endured the trauma of the transplant. Fortunately, Friend's personality resonated with Felicia. "We've found the quintessential sage mother," she said, "the wise aunt we all wish we had to referee family arguments."

The despondence Felicia voiced in those first sessions echoed the experience of Melissa Fernandez, another CGD mom whose marriage suffered after her son Rocco made it home to Louisiana after his Duke transplant. "I was so unhappy. I was so beaten down, I had nothing left. I didn't know who I was anymore." Trying to reclaim their old selves, Melissa and her husband went on their first date in years. It didn't go well. "At dinner, he seemed the same, but I knew I was different. I said, 'I think I want a divorce. I can't do this anymore.'"

Her husband insisted they work on it; Melissa says they went to a couple of counseling sessions. "But I still had that anger. I picked fights, we fought about everything. Big stuff, small stuff. I would yell, scream, and curse. He would just listen and try to explain his side. But I didn't *want* to hear his side. I was angry at the world."

My anger was on a comeback tour of its own. I wasn't losing my temper every ten minutes—my Program had modulated outward expressions of rage—but it was on a constant slow boil.

I felt cheated. This was the phase of our lives where we were supposed to be catching up with renewed vigor and focus to the peers who'd been getting ahead for the past five years without the burdens of a rare disease diagnosis. I wanted us to be like that guy in *Chariots of Fire* who comes back to win the 400 meters after someone knocks him to the turf at the first turn. Instead it now looked like we'd never get past the PWASK state—like an immunodeficient baby whose body spends its energy fighting infection instead of growing, we'd always be struggling just to keep our shit together, stuck in place like a crackhead I once saw at Grand Central amusing himself by methodically walking up the down escalator.

The sense of social unbelonging ramped up, metastasizing from an undifferentiated walking-on-the-moon feeling of foreignness into an acute antagonism toward the lives of the healthy and their contemptible trivialities. Of course, even the happiest people are often coping with (or masking) serious problems, but in my blazing misanthropy all I saw was naive bliss. In my mind these people were the Whos of Whoville, and they were everywhere—at the gym, the office, social media—humblebragging about every marginally impressive experience or achievement, hopelessly addicted to electronic stimulus, corrupting every business email with fraudulent exclamation points, complaining about the slightest discomfiture as if it were a plague of locusts, obsessively optimizing every facet of their lives like Scientologists.

I was sick and tired of being sick and tired. I was sad and angry about being sad and angry. I didn't fit in, nor did I much want to.

John Boyle said these tales of alienation and resentment are common. He compared them to accounts of returning combat vets. "Obviously being in a war zone is more intense and dangerous, but on the flip side, most people will self-censor when they are around soldiers who just came home. They get it. With us, most of our scars are semi-private, and not everyone understands what our experience is all about."

The life-affirming Facebook posts ceased. Escape fantasies shouldered their way into my daydreams. A one-way ticket to Moldova or some other country with no extradition treaty. Stealing someone's identity and disappearing into a new life aboard a Great Lakes freighter. A blowout party in Goa followed by an extended sabbatical in the Mumbai slums like the dude in *Shantaram*. Joining the priesthood and leading a parish in the Central African Republic. Dealing drugs, teaching high school, or perhaps both, in Barrow, Alaska. Or maybe a simple relocation back to Mom's house. Just get me out of here.

Periods of de facto marital separation punctuated the following months—separate beds, silent treatments—but we stuck to our agreement: shrinks before lawyers. It may have been delusional or arrogant or patriarchal, but I believed that even at my worst, my kids were better off with a messed-up father in the house than with none.

I was certainly better off with them. My moments of happiness, when they happened, were built almost exclusively around the kids' joys and achievements, a case study in the perils of vicarious living. Of these moments there was none greater than the first day of school, attendance at which had been Sebastian's true Make-A-Wish since he'd first seen his sister walk out the front door with a backpack years earlier. His scalp and hair issue had stabilized enough not to elicit comment, and he'd bounced back from his Canadian fever. The Tuesday after Labor Day, we joined our neighbors walking with the kids to school, Sebastian with a new Thomas the Tank Engine backpack slung over his narrow shoulders, beaming with pride. This was all he'd ever wanted.

The kid had spent fifteen of the prior eighteen months in some form of strict quarantine. Questions about his socialization abounded. We wondered if he would be scared to say goodbye to Mommy and Daddy and walk into class by himself. He wasn't. We wondered if he was going to be bullied as the smallest kid in his class. He wasn't. We wondered if he'd have trouble making friends. He didn't. We wondered if sending him into the petri dish of a kindergarten classroom with a one-year-old's immune system—the equivalent of South Korean soldiers training barechested in the snow—would put him at risk for infection.

It did.

Between Thanksgiving and Easter, he contracted a string of sicknesses that bordered on the Dickensian. In order: pneumonia, croup, the flu, and shingles. The last was particularly ghastly—an angry red reptilian rash that snaked from his left knee up around to his lower back. The agony reduced him to a state of quiet whimpering, prostrate on Felicia's lap, re-creating the pietàs I'd witnessed so often pre-transplant. "It's awful to watch him suffer," she said as she strapped him into his car seat for a doctor's visit, "but he's so stoic, after all he's been through." He collapsed once in the back of the Subaru, pale as a sheet, and though the doctors kept him out of the hospital with a battery of prescriptions, he ended up missing more than a month of school.

It was a dark winter. The cumulative stress was wearing us down and tearing us apart. Felicia could get overprescriptive and preachy. For her part, Lydia began resenting all the extra attention and what she perceived as favoritism directed at her little brother. Her perpetually sunny personality clouded over with recurring tantrums and chronic back talk, especially toward her mother. And, as a crowning achievement, through a combination of bad attitude and burnout I managed to lose my job. I spent much of the winter panicking over how I was going to provide for the family and pay the eternal influx of medical bills we seemed destined to accrue. On garbage day mornings, I resumed my habit of gazing wistfully out the window at the miracle of trash pickup, wishing the same burly group of men could scoop up the rest of our troubles and make them just . . . go away.

Clearly, I'd neglected my Program and the consequences had been disastrous. I was wrong to think I'd be fine so long as my son was—*my* health was an entirely separate matter. As I bounced off rock bottom, I called on my friend Dan Harris and one of his teachers, the renowned meditation expert Sharon Salzberg, for help. They kindly carved out time for me, and our special sits probably staved off a full-blown nervous breakdown, but what he said was true: mindfulness works much better as prophylaxis than as a Band-Aid.

We'd never imagined tripping and falling so hard *after* we'd crossed the finish line, but that's how it played out. We'd been dealt more than we could handle and the future of our family was in doubt. "You can't count on a Hollywood ending," said John Boyle. "It's really more like *Into the Woods*—the first act is traditional fairy tale stuff. The second act is what happens afterward. There's some beauty . . . and there's some horror.

"It's just a fact—the results lay out on a bell curve. Not everybody makes it."

Chapter 19

A Dog Named Hope

She was the skankiest dog in the shelter.

A mutt. Half Chihuahua, half who knows what—corgi, Jack Russell, dachshund, or maybe daddy was just another mutt. She had oversized ears, the left of which had been bitten or cut in some peculiar manner to leave a narrow jigsaw piece of flesh missing on its top edge. Her coat, similar to the markings of a Holstein cow, was ravaged by hairless patches of pink, poxed flesh around the neck and tummy, caused by allergy and/or infection. And she was jittery—her walnut-sized canine brain knew enough to realize she was in a bad place and that, compared to the other candidates in the adjacent cages, she didn't stand much of a chance in a beauty contest where first prize was escape.

I'd come under protest. Yes, we'd promised Sebastian we could get a dog after he made it home from transplant and Dr. Prasad had given his blessing. But as much as I knew anything, I knew our family could not take on another long-term responsibility, especially not one who looked like this much trouble. I peered into her eyes and saw a future of feces, fleas, and fights over mounting vet bills. She might not look like much of a threat, but I smelled it on her: this eleven-pound mongrel would be the final fracture. She would shatter our family for good.

"Her name's Hope," Lydia said, pointing to a handwritten cardboard square affixed to the door of the cage. It was our daughter who, after being overpowered during the mandatory test walk by a hyper Lab-beagle mix I'd suggested first, had gravitated toward this pen. Sebastian followed and, like his sister, fell in love at first sight.

"She's a perfect fit for us," mused Felicia as she bent down to let the dog sniff her hand. "Sick, scarred, and scared." My wife had long been part of the pro-pet lobby; on the Unit, she'd reiterated her assurance to Sebastian that a dog would be the reward for his heroism.

The staffers at the shelter swore that after a month of prescription meds Hope's hair would grow back. *Daily meds and hair loss,* I thought, *that sounds familiar.* They said we could give her any name we chose—"Hope" had been assigned arbitrarily just four days earlier by the driver who'd transported her and a dozen other rescues from central Ohio.

"We'll take her as is," I said, settling into a space of fatalistic acquiescence as familiar as the discolored cushions of our TV-room couch. I made just one iron-clad demand—that Felicia and the kids sign a contract I drew up, acknowledging that I would be responsible for absolutely none of the animal's care and feeding.

A series of pleasant surprises ensued. The kids not only signed the contract, they honored it. The doggie medicine worked. The hair grew back.

Most of all, Hope proved me dead wrong. She didn't yip, she didn't tear up the house, she didn't even want to be walked. Truth be told, she was as low-maintenance as a cat.

Above all, she immediately emerged as a radiant presence in our lives, a being who seemed to exist for no other purpose than to give and receive love. Never angry, never aloof—a constant source of joy in an ever-expanding universe of entropy and indifference. In short, she was just what we needed. I was never happier to be wrong.

My miscalculation was precisely this: after five and a half years focusing obsessively on our own problems and issues, the countless crises real and imagined, what we needed above all was to direct our attentions outside our little circle, to be providers of charity for once instead of receivers.

Hope (the dog) was the start of it. Before I found a new TV job I spent some time helping out at a local soup kitchen; once I went back to work, I volunteered to teach Sunday school. (I still wasn't convinced God existed, but I was convinced the stories of Christianity were beautiful enough to pass on.) Limited though the commitment was, just spending a little time each week focusing on kids other than ours was like snapping out of a trance. The weird universal father feelings I continued to have while practicing loving-kindness could be put to some respectable use.

My giving back efforts were a trifle compared to Felicia's. She'd already been involved with the Immune Deficiency Foundation and the CGD community prior to Sebastian's transplant, but as her daily obligations with Sebastian's medical needs evaporated, she threw herself into patient advocacy and research with a passion. "I can't just go back to regular life, worrying about what brand of paper towels to buy, without helping others with what I've learned," she told me. "I know how much I relied on other mothers who helped me, who were there for me, and told me I wasn't alone." With the encouragement of Dr. Malech at the NIH, she ended up launching the CGD Association of America. Today she devotes much of her time reaching out to other moms to hear their stories, offer the best support and advice available, and share the latest research. For all my pooh-poohing of her faith-based view of life, of the two of us she's become by far the more fluent in the details of current medical science and treatment options.

She's even become part of the research herself. Back at NIH, Dr. Malech and his colleagues are interested increasingly in the immune functions of not just CGD patients but also the carriers—the moms with the recessive mutated X chromosome. These women, warriors fighting for their children and their families, sadly also suffer from diminished neutrophil function and are susceptible to CGD-type infections. Many deal with chronic fatigue, arthritis, and trouble concentrating. "It's not something you necessarily see, but it's something you feel," says Felicia. In their tireless crusade against the unknown, the NIH researchers have invited Felicia—and her mother, the oldest living CGD carrier on record—down to the fortified campus in Bethesda to participate in tests and studies, treating them as needed, while hoping to unlock more of the immune system's secrets. "If we study enough of the carriers," Malech explained, "we may be able to understand just how many cells you really need to be protected from infection." There's also data suggesting CGD carriers have lower rates of some heart diseases and cancers—it is hypothesized that their overcompensating immune systems may hold the key to the prevention of those common killers.

All of the above gave us a greater sense of purpose, perspective, and peace. But it would be unfair to deny proper credit to the simple passage of time. With time, Sebastian's hair grew back, he climbed into the 50th percentile on the growth curve, and his acquired immune system caught up with those of his peers. Aside from a daily multivitamin, today he takes no medicine. There have been corresponding cutbacks in our Purell budget, though we will continue to press elevator buttons with our knuckles for the rest of our lives.

The only noticeable difference between Sebastian and his classmates is social—compensating for years without friends, he can be excessively huggy and attached to a designated BFF. It's heartbreaking when other kids are put off by that, but presumably he'll outgrow his tendency to love too much and learn to respect "appropriate" boundaries. In other words, to conform. Oh well.

With time, our stressed prefrontal cortexes began their own long recoveries. Fortunately, as much as post-traumatic stress is real, so is post-traumatic growth. "The rodent data suggests that with time spent in a nonstressed state, the gray matter restores," Dr. Arnsten told me. "But it also suggests you haven't forgotten about the horrible thing, whatever it is, and you have a lower threshold to retrigger a stress response. It takes a long time for the brain to recover fully. About as long as it takes to shrink." If that holds true for us, we should return to our pre-crisis brain state sometime in the summer of 2024, presuming our lives remain stress free.

Even if they don't—a fair bet—we're now more confident we can manage whatever comes, not only because we're ready to pray, meditate, medicate, work out, and get therapy on a constant or as-needed basis, but because we've learned to recognize the stress response for what it is—an old, annoying relative—and to lean into its presence to the degree we are able. We now regard stress and anxiety much the way Nietzsche regarded his chronic stomach pain: "I have given a name to my pain and call it 'dog,'" he wrote. "It is just as faithful, just as obtrusive and shameless, just as entertaining, just as clever as any other dog." Let it be thus: we call our dog Hope and we call our stress Dog. A pair of loyal pets.

We've negotiated a truce with our sense of unbelonging too. It will never fully dissipate, and that's okay. Our experience has put us out of step with mainstream opinion on countless fronts, but we cannot unsee what we saw. It will remain popular to bad-mouth the American health care system and its obscene affordability issues without acknowledging its redeeming qualities; after seeing people flock from around the world to partake of its fruits, we will not be among them. It will remain obligatory to denounce the depredations of Big Pharma; after watching its innovations—from vaccines to fentanyl—save so many young lives, we cannot join the chorus. It will remain fashionable to sound alarms about the perceived dangers of genetically modified organisms, but how can we be part of the torches-and-pitchforks mob when our son *is* a GMO? The long-term effects of his chimerism cannot be predicted—his complexion has turned a more latte shade than he was before, and we expect other quirky surprises down the road—but without the transplanters' "unnatural" meddling, he'd still be imprisoned in his disease. Or dead.

The marriage? After a full year of additional therapy, we're hanging in there. Ferguson was right: a short-term commitment was never going to work. Full disclosure—our relationship can be boring; it can be boisterous; and the D-word, that reliable tear gas canister, still gets shot into the air if we disobey Ferguson's commandments for long. Our parenting philosophies diverge enough for the kids to try to play us off each other, and my skeptical/empiricist sensibility still collides periodically with Felicia's assertive approach to spirituality and her New Age proclivities. (She once scalded my face tenderly applying essential oils she'd neglected to dilute. A classic Lucy-Desi scene ensued.)

That said, no one's going anywhere. By now we're less husband and wife than two halves of the same person, welded together by the acetylene torch of a parenting experience no one else can ever fully understand. And, as with the *Clockwork Orange* reaction we developed to on-screen violence, I now get a crippling nausea in the aftermath of any marital discord. If we fight, I'm soon groveling for forgiveness to make the feeling go away.

We knew we'd come full circle when Lydia performed "Home" at one of her piano recitals—the Phillip Phillips acoustic hit that charted back in 2012 at the time of Sebastian's diagnosis. We'd listened to it tearfully back in our Manhattan apartment as we held our fragile, stricken baby, and its uplifting lyrics about fighting demons and fear led Felicia to feel almost like it had been written for us. "To see our beautiful daughter playing the same song years later was one of the most moving experiences of my life," she said. We took family photos under a tree outside the recital hall and, locking eyes, my wife and I renewed our wedding vows in silence.

All the other couples we met are sticking with it too. At least so far. The Fernandez family, the Hickses, the Assells, and the Richelses are still together, while down in Florida, Stacy Ayers reports: "Our marriage is fine. [My husband] jokes about it all the time. He understands that I'm crazy, but he respects that if I bring up some medical concern at least it's been researched."

Susan and Keith Morrow may express it best. "We always fight, but we always come back to the kid," said Susan. "If we're fighting and Keith is on the couch that night, he still knows he has to go and check on Evelyn first thing in the morning. Kids with her condition die in their sleep all the time. Keith doesn't ever want me to be the one to find her."

Susan paused. "But some days, I really do fucking hate you, hon."

"Yeah," Keith said with a sigh. "I know you do."

Three years out from transplant, all the kids we met who made it home are still alive, though the Morrows don't know how long they will have with Evelyn. Like any Hurler syndrome patient, the transplant bought her time but not a cure. As the Morrows wait and lobby for new medicine and new treatments to come on line, Evelyn is enjoying the arrival of a new baby sister, Henrietta (named after Henrietta Lacks). Susan is optimistic, but realistic. "I'm going to be happy if Evelyn makes it to fourteen. I think that's when it's going to really start to go downhill for us. And I don't know if we'll stay married if she dies. I might just blame everybody but myself and get divorced."

The faith journeys of these families have varied dramatically. The Ayerses became even more devout and Stacy continues to praise the Lord on Facebook at every opportunity. Susan Morrow says she oscillates in and out of piety in an inverse relationship to Evelyn's health—the better the kid is doing, the less she calls on God. And Melissa Fernandez has abandoned her faith altogether—Rocco is thriving, but after his transplant, she lost another child in utero. "It has broken me completely. And the only reason I keep going is Rocco. He gives me that little bit of hope, but God has given me way more than I can handle."

Conversely, the parents of Khaleda Assell, the fourteen-year-old who died on the Unit, say their faith is what's kept them together and capable of moving forward. "You never fully recover," says Amanda. "Something will hit you, feelings come back and it's a deep sadness that you'd not want anyone to feel; sometimes we'll see things like her best friend driving and we'll be, like, 'OMG, Khaleda would have been doing that.' It's crushing. But then we'll cross paths with people close to her, and they'll remind us how she changed their lives. At least we got to have the time with her that we did."

Every spring, Dr. Kurtzberg and the Duke PBMT Program host the Rainbow of Heroes Walk to raise funds for the family support program. It is as much a reunion for patients and their families as a fundraiser, and the year we made it down we had the chance to thank Kurtzberg and some of the other staffers in person. Many elements of the event are what you'd expect—bright T-shirts, balloons, bouncy houses, a wall with photos of all the transplanted kids, inspiring speeches, an abundance of hugs. What surprised us was the large turnout of parents of kids who *hadn't* survived. Their tragic outcomes notwithstanding, something about the Duke experience, the intensity of the love and care they'd felt there, continued to exert a centripetal force on their lives. A few couples had even moved to Durham permanently, just to stay close to that warmth.

The special vibe was, in part, what led our dear friend Tina Merrill to redirect her own life. After seeing what we went through, and the immense difference she made for us, she says she felt a transformative sense of fulfillment. "Helping people in such dire need," she said, "you have a unique opportunity to give real comfort and assistance. Some people think you need to be working for the Gates Foundation to make a difference in the world, but it's possible to have a profound impact on an intimate scale." After we went home, Tina quit her COO job at a Durham software company and became a nurse at Duke University Hospital.

Sebastian is still drawn to Duke too. Barely old enough to retain long-term memory of his time in North Carolina, he snaps at any opportunity to go back (we returned again for Nurse Liz's wedding, at which he was a guest of honor). He spends every moment of these visits frolicking like Durham is an amusement park.

On the weekend of the Rainbow of Heroes Walk we paid a visit to Unit 5200. Some kids come out of transplant terrified of doctors and hospitals. Sebastian had shown a remarkable toughness to date, enduring all his post-transplant immunizations with little more than a clenched jaw and fist, but we didn't know how he'd react. Enough time had passed that we'd forgotten the sequence of the hygiene routine and had to follow the written instructions on the wall of the antechamber. But once we peeked inside room 5214, vacant at the time, all the sense memory returned. Our old friends were right where we'd left them— the vitals monitor; the urine jug; the tiny couch bed; and of course the noble pole, standing at attention, awaiting its next tour of duty.

Sebastian, his budding sense of humor recognizing an opening, broke the silence—"Hey, Mommy, I want *another* transplant!" If that's how the kid thinks back on his experience, someone must have done something right.

We may never see that Unit again—a new PBMTU is under construction as of this writing. Dr. Prasad assures me its rooms will be bigger and the parents' sleeping arrangements more commodious, but that will likely be the least of the advances. The revolutions in transplant technique, immunology, and gene therapies are not only proceeding but accelerating. Dr. Prasad reports that in the few years since we were at Duke the population of leukemia patients has dropped because so many are now opting for the new CAR T-cell therapy instead of transplant. Meanwhile, new research is making cord blood transplant a viable option for new classes of patients and diseases. Kurtzberg is years into her trial using cord blood as a treatment for neurological disorders like cerebral palsy and autism. "It's showing encouraging results," she told me. "Though it's not a transplant, it's an infusion, using the patient's own cells as a fancy drug. We're trying to figure out if it works, and if so, why it works." Discovering a cure for autism, the disease that first attracted Kurtzberg to medicine, would be a fitting final achievement for her legendary career.

At the NIH and elsewhere, gene therapy trials are yielding astonishing results with a variety of genetic disorders. To name but one example, a year after we made it home from Duke, the FDA approved the first gene therapy for an inherited disease, a form of congenital blindness called inherited retinal degeneration. In short, they're curing the blind.

"Since the Renaissance many people have felt like they are living in a special time," says Dr. Malech, "but this much is true: in my career I've seen exponential changes in treatment and care, and I can now see the light at the end of the tunnel where improvements in transplant and gene therapy are bringing us to a place where we'll be able to offer truly curative treatments for a whole host of disorders. Even to me as a scientist, it just seems miraculous."

Ah, the M-word. If Dr. Malech is throwing it around, perhaps we should all get on board with Freeman Dyson and concede that God exists, and that science and technology are his greatest gifts. For those looking to reconcile the spiritual and scientific, that may be the best way to thread the needle.

Catholicism is my religion, but science will always be my faith. I offered my son up to modern medicine like a little Isaac, and my trust was rewarded. As I recall, it was E. O. Wilson who remarked that today's scientists should be revered the way shamans and witch doctors were by ancient tribes. It is fact, borne out by the COVID-19 crisis, that many of today's real heroes—the ones saving lives—are unglamorous and self-effacing people who spend their days reading charts and peering into microscopes. And in my experience, their big brains don't crowd out their hearts—upon reviewing Sebastian's medical records I came across a random note from a pediatric cardiologist who only saw him once, in those anguished pre-diagnosis months. In the summary of his findings he included a personal addendum to the pediatrician, a casual remark I was never supposed to see but which touched me deeply nonetheless: "Thank you for referring this beautiful infant for consultation."

On Saturday, October 6, 2018, almost six years to the day after the diagnosis, it was time to take off the training wheels.

Sebastian strapped on his helmet and I put the leash on Hope as we prepared to walk the little red bike down to the nearby schoolyard. Donning a hoodie, I caught a glimpse of myself in the living room mirror and did a double take. Brimming with restored energy and excitement, I felt like Lord Byron; the reflection staring back looked more like the Ancient Mariner. My upper eyelids had begun to droop, the lower ones puffed like tea bags. My head, once crowned with a salad of Bacchian curls, was now almost entirely barren on top and perfectly gray on the sides. My stubble was snow, as was a creeping percentage of my eyebrows. This was not the face of a young man.

Compensation for such a wizening countenance, one might presuppose, should be hard-earned wisdom. Like Joseph Campbell's archetypal hero, had I not been called reluctantly on a journey, struggled through a netherworld of challenges, and now returned to share the sacred knowledge those struggles had yielded? And is this not the moment where a dutiful reader has a right to expect a payout in the form of transcendent, been-to-the-mountaintop life lessons?

I'm afraid much of what we learned is little more than self-help clichés: we've learned to take responsibility for our own behavior, regardless of what excuse extreme circumstance may provide; we are grateful for the little things; we've been emancipated from the tyranny of conspicuous consumption and the mandates of the parenting industrial complex; we have a healthier sense of proportion; we embrace our imperfections and vulnerabilities; and we believe that pursuits of happiness are secondary to pursuits of meaning. Living thus, we've tried to build a better immune system for our minds and souls, protecting them as best we can from a world of constant assault and pollution, striving to remain true to our natural nobility. We now have the freedom to indulge some of our desires and whims—vacations can be fun—but we've learned there is no higher freedom than living in accordance with the laws you make for yourself.

Still, the most powerful lessons were the simplest ones, the ones I should have internalized as a kid, long before the stern education purchased with six years of parenting on the edge. At least now I could pass them on to my son. Hopefully, he wouldn't have to learn the hard way. Happily, they applied to the challenge of riding a bike without training wheels as much as to life's other little tests.

On the schoolyard asphalt I held the seat and handlebars steady as his six-year-old cerebellum gradually got with the program. He wobbled, he fell, his eyes welled with tears of frustration. He insisted he wasn't ready, we should wait another year. All the while, I repeated the few grains of wisdom I'd been able to tweeze out of our ordeal.

> *It's okay to be scared.*
> *You're not the first person to go through this.*
> *Be patient.*
> *Focus on what's in front of you.*
> *Push forward.*
> *Protect your head.*
> *Hold on.*
> *You can do this.*

After twenty minutes of failure his spine straightened, the handlebars steadied, the self-doubt disappeared. With one final balancing boost I jogged beside the bike as he began pedaling and, once released, circumnavigated the schoolyard. His quavering *"Daaddeee . . ."* changed from a timid SOS into an exultant imperative that I bear witness to his new power and independence: *"Daddy! Look!"*

Hope barked encouragement as he came around and took a second lap, leaving me behind. I inhaled the future and thought of the countless people who'd labored, given, and suffered to make this happen. Thanks to them, our child has a lifetime of paths before him to explore and conquer, some with us, many more without. Whether his ambitions turn out Olympian or prosaic, he is free to pursue them without fear. A parent can ask for nothing more.

Is it okay if we just leave it at that?

Acknowledgments

The trouble with thanking the people who've helped accomplish a project of any size are the inevitable errors of omission. Forgive me in advance for the many that are about to follow.

First, my wife, Felicia, to whom I am infinitely indebted for her tireless caregiving for Sebastian and our family. She was just as devoted to the completion of this book, sharing journals she kept throughout Sebastian's transplant and recovery. Those first-person accounts, especially of moments I missed, were vital to the narrative. Her editing and fact-checking skills were equally invaluable.

Many others sustained us through our "journey," starting with our families: my mother, Marta Zamora; my father, Mike Sancho, and his wife, Bridget Shirley; my sister, Victoria Sancho Lobis, and her husband, Seth Lobis; my cousins Lee and Colin England, Robert and Alba DeMarea, and Isabel Garcia-Amador, Federico Amador, and Federico Zamora, to name but a few; Felicia's mother, Barbara Morton, and her deceased father, Howard; her cousins Tina, Harry, and Elena Itameri. A long list of friends including but not limited to: Fred Pincombe, Elizabeth Chakkapan, Carley Foreman, Jenny Davidson, Amy Davidson Sorkin, Chris Wiedemann, Danielle Bregman, Ty Alevizos, Caleb Hellerman, Kamran Atabai, Mark Gimbel, Alex Friedman, Bruno Maddox, Adam Lehner, Luke Barr, Yumi Moriwaki, Tanya Selvaratnam, Jonathan Sigel, Tony Verderosa, Jen Braunschweiger, Betty Ng, Sam Brown, Natasha Shaprio, Bruno Kavanaugh, Jake and Maya Phipps, and Khakasa Wapenyi, who passed in 2013. Cherished former colleagues and mentors including David Sloan, Jessica Velmans, Lisa Soloway, Danielle Rossen, Matt Lombardi, Terri Lichstein, Janice Johnston, Andrew Papparella, Marc Dorian, Jim Dubreuil, Ed Lopez, Gail Deutsch, Claire Weinraub, Chris Cuomo, Elizabeth Vargas,

Acknowledgments

Jeanmarie Condon, Tom Sibrowski, James Goldston, Kerry Smith, Nicole Gallagher, John Zucker, Davis Townsend, Jon Meyersohn, Chris Kilmer, Jazmine Garner, David Doss, Al Prieto, Lauren Brennan, Caroline Welch, Matt Gutman, Mollie Auran, Sun Min, Josh Gelman, Susan Zirinsky, and Al Briganti. And of course, the core of our local support system during transplant—Tina Merrill Buchwalter, Jessica Tang, and Hunter Glass. All of the above provided much-needed support, love (including tough love), and guidance.

The following charities also deserve recognition and support: the Ronald McDonald Houses, the Duke Family Support Program, the Children's Organ Transplant Association, Hayden's Journey of Inspiration, the Immune Deficiency Foundation, Be the Match, the Make-A-Wish Foundation, Angel Flight, and the CGD Association of America, which Felicia now runs.

As for the book itself, my deepest thanks go to Dan Harris, who supported this project from proposal to completion; the inimitable Luke Janklow and Claire Dippel at Janklow & Nesbit; and my editor, Caroline Sutton, along with Hannah Steigmeyer and the rest of the outstanding team at Avery. It takes courage to get behind a first manuscript from an unknown author, and just as much effort and patience to make sure it ends up good for more than lining birdcages.

I was fortunate to have a bounty of material to work with—troves of medical records, personal emails, texts, and social media posts. Still, I would have been lost without the generous contributions of the people who agreed to be interviewed and contribute their recollections, wisdom, and intensely personal stories. These include other patient parents Melissa Layman Fernandez, Justine Richels, Dawn Adams, Stacey Ayers, Susan and Keith Morrow, Patty Furco, Travis and Luanne Hicks, and Amanda Assell. For sharing their vast medical knowledge and precious time (as well as saving our son's life), I am also indebted to the following outstanding medical professionals: Dr. Vinod Prasad, Dr. Joanne Kurtzberg, Dr. Suhag Parikh, Dr. Harry Malech, Dr. Ronit Herzog, Dr. Gary Edelstein; nurses

Acknowledgments

Liz Vaughn, Katie Burke, Bobbie Caraher, Marybeth Tetlow, and Jenna Boyd; and LCSW Lindsay Gallo. Two of our marriage counselors, William Lent and Robert Ferguson, also agreed to be interviewed and to share their notes from our sessions. My apologies for making them relive those experiences.

Lastly, a final salute to the patients—of both rare and common diseases—who've had it tougher than we did, especially those who didn't make it. My son—and frankly everyone alive today thanks to modern medicine—stands at the peak of a mountain built through their suffering and sacrifice. Now and forever, their breath is one with ours.

Index

Page numbers followed by "n" indicate notes.

Index

Index

CRISPR revolution, 69
Crossan, John Dominic, 40, 200, 267
CT scans, 120, 122–23, 133, 136, 143,
    151, 230, 249, 264
Curlin pump, home infusion, 234–35
cyclosporine, 190, 210, 239, 270,
    271, 277
cystic fibrosis (CF) patients, xvi–xvii
cytomegalovirus, 216
Cytoxan, 160, 169

Dagestan ethnic conflicts, 179
"Daisy Cutter" Air Force bomb, 178
Dakin, Henry, and Dakin's solution, 64
Dangerfield, Rodney, 200, 211
Dawn, 79–80
dealing with what's in front of you, 48,
    83, 170, 258, 295
dendrites and stress, 50, 276
depression in rare-disease families, xi,
    32, 85, 207, 256
Designated Survivor (TV show), 250
"designer" baby for transplant,
    79–80
diagnosis of CGD, 4, 19–20, 32–39,
    43, 46, 52, 59, 67, 74, 228, 255,
    263, 288
diaper rash, 22, 23
diet for transplants, 161–62, 207, 229
diphtheria eradication, 32
discharge from PBMTU, 150, 193–94,
    215–19, 221–32, 257
DNA, 47, 69, 70, 161, 181, 190
    See also chimerism
doctor burnout, 187–88
dog (Hope), 234, 269, 283–85, 287,
    293, 295
donor search, 75–80, 104, 108, 128, 136,
    152, 160, 165, 177–78, 180, 196
dopamine, 49, 85, 207
double income no kids (DINKs), 11
double transplants, UCB, 106, 173, 177

Duke Children's Hospital, 115, 119,
    120–21, 123, 154, 216, 235
    See also Pediatric Blood and Marrow
    Transplant Unit (PBMTU)
Duke Gardens, 235
Duke Life Flight crash, 213–14
Duke University Hospital, x, xiii, 4–5,
    104, 108, 291
    See also Pediatric Blood and Marrow
    Transplant Unit (PBMTU)
dying with dignity, 196–97
Dyson, Freeman, 243, 293

E. coli, 162
Eastwood, Clint, 14, 203
ECG, 19
ECMO, 194
Edelstein, Gary, 16, 17, 19, 22–23, 26,
    38, 93
emotional detachment of parents, 21
England, Lee, 56, 58, 64
engraftment, 61, 62, 63, 106, 136, 155,
    165, 172–73, 186, 192–93, 204–6,
    208–13, 215, 216, 217, 218, 221,
    248, 265
environmental threats, 58, 83–84, 85,
    86–87, 89
epidemiology, xiv
Epstein-Barr virus, 62, 144
ethnic groups and matched unrelated
    donors, 76, 77, 106
expulsion from Ronald McDonald
    House, xi, 134–36

Facebook, 45, 82, 96–97, 102, 130, 149,
    150, 207, 218, 227, 250, 255, 267,
    280, 290
fatal granulomatous disease, 59
    See also chronic granulomatous
    disease (CGD)
FDA, 60, 69, 70, 75, 142, 292

Index

Index

Index

Index

Index